Attention Deficit Disorder

*A Concise Source of Information
for Parents and Teachers*

2nd Edition, Revised and Expanded

H. Moghadam, M.D.

&

Joel Fagan, M.D.

Detselig Enterprises Ltd.
Calgary, Alberta, Canada

Attention Deficit Disorder
© 1988, 1994 H. Moghadam & Joel Fagan. All rights reserved.
Published 1988. 2nd edition 1994.

H. Moghadam, MD, MPH, FRCPC
Emeritus Professor of Pediatrics and Community Health
Sciences, University of Calgary, Consulting Pediatrician,
Alberta Children's Hospital: Calgary, ALB

J. Fagan, MD FRCPC, MSc
Professor of Pediatrics, University of Calgary
Director, Developmental Clinic, Alberta Children's Hospital

With contributions by:

S. Gupta, EdD
Psychologist, Alberta Children's Hospital

M. Haug, PhD
Clinical Pyschologist, Alberta Children's Hospital

C. McFee, MSW, Social Worker
Former staff of Alberta Children's Hospital

C. Garbet-Smith, MSW, Social Worker
Alberta Children's Hospital

Canadian Cataloguing in Publication Data

Moghadam, H. (Hossein)
  Attention deficit disorder

  ISBN 1-55059-082-0

  1. Attention-deficit hyperactivity disorder. 2. Hyperactive
children. I. Fagan, Joel. II. Title.
RJ506.H9M63 1994   618.92'8589   C94-910884-7

Detselig Enterprises Ltd.
210, 1220 Kensington Rd. N.W.
Calgary, Alberta   T2N 3P5   Canada

Detselig Enterprises Ltd. appreciates the financial support for our 1994 publishing program, provided by the Department of Canadian Heritage, Canada Council and the Alberta Foundation for the Arts, a beneficiary of the Lottery Fund of the Government of Alberta.

Cover drawing and interior art by Heather Sawyer
Cover Design by Dean MacDonald

Printed in Canada   ISBN 1-55059-082-0   SAN 115-0324

*This book is dedicated to the parents and teachers
of hyperactive and other misunderstood children*

A Disclaimer

This book is a concise source of information on attention deficit disorder, and as such does not attempt to completely cover this complicated, and at times, controversial topic. Although every attempt has been made to discuss the principal aspects of what is currently understood about this topic, the brevity of the presentation has precluded the inclusion of every detail. This book is not intended to be a substitute for your physician's advice. Every child with attention deficit disorder is a unique individual, and his/her management should be individually designed in keeping with the particular circumstances of the child, family, and classroom teacher. Neither the authors, nor the publisher accept any legal or moral responsibility, nor any liability, for actions taken by parents which are contrary to the advice of their physician.

Brand names of medications have been included in the book because, normally, parents and teachers are not familiar with the drugs' generic names. This is not to be construed, however, as an endorsement or a criticism of these or other products. Statements regarding the therapeutic properties, the effectiveness, and the side effects of drugs are based entirely on the authors' experience and may differ from the experience of other physicians.

Acknowledgements

The authors and contributors wish to thank Ms. Rosanne Fortini-Burrows for her patience and tolerance during the preparation of the first edition of this book, and Mrs. Joy Bilozir for her expert word processing skills during the writing of this second edition.

We wish to also thank Dr. Bonnie Kaplan, Director of the Behavioral Research Unit at the Alberta Children's Hospital. Her reviewing of several chapters of this book, practical comments and suggestions were a tremendous help and are sincerely appreciated.

We are also grateful to Heather Sawyer for her illustrations which appear in this book.

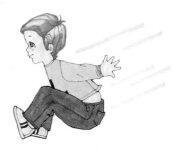

Contents

Preface   **9**

Chapter 1   A Brief Historical Review   **13**

Chapter 2   ADD – What is it?   **17**

Chapter 3   The Prevalence of ADD   **25**

Chapter 4   The Possible Causes   **27**

Brain Damage   28
Biochemical Brain Malfunction   29
Genetic Influences   29
Infection   30
Maturation Lag   30
Poisons   31
Hormone Abnormalities   31
Sensitivity to Fluorescent Light   32
Food Sensitivity   32
Summary   32

Chapter 5   Diagnosis   **35**

Diagnostic Criteria for Attention-Deficit-
Hyperactivity Disorder (ADHD)   36
Criteria for the Severity of ADHD   38
History   38
Parent Questionnaire   40
Teacher Questionnaire   42
Commonly Reported Behavior Patterns   45
Medical Examination   48
Psychological Tests   49
Hair Analysis   50
Allergy Tests   51

Chapter 6   Management: Drug Therapy   53

    Stimulant Therapy   54
    Drug Trials   56
    Questions about Stimulant Drugs   58

Chapter 7   Behavior Management   73

    Behavior Modification   73
    Use of Behavior Modification   75
    Limitations of Behavior Therapy   77
    Acquisition of Self-Control   79
    Cognative Behavior Therapy   80
    Social Skills Training   81

Chapter 8   Parental and Family Issues   83

    Common Concerns and Problems   83
    Self-Esteem Issues   84
    The Effects of the ADD Child on the Family .   84
    The Effects of External Forces on the Family .   86
    Parents' Reactions to the Diagnosis   87
    Coping with the Problem   88
    Parental Burn Out   89
    Seeking Help and Meeting Professionals . . .   90
    Resources for Parents and Families   91

Chapter 9   Classroom Management   97

    Classroom Problems   98
    Cognative Behavior Therapy   102

Chapter 10   Other Approaches to Management   107

    Diet and Hyperactivity   107
    Sugar and Hyperactivity   111
    Megavitamin Therapy   112

Chapter 11   ADD in Adolescence   115

    Adolescents with ADD   116
    Treatment for the Adolescent with ADD . . .   117
    The Newly Diagnosed Adolescent   119

Chapter 12   When ADD Children Grow Up   121

    Outcome Studies   121

Preface

It has now been six years since the first edition of this book was published. Since that time interest in children with attention deficit disorder has continued to increase among parents, teachers and other professionals. More physicians, psychologists school counsellors and others are aware of the problems and special needs of these children. Nevertheless, many children continue to underachieve academically, and to experience conflict and disappointment in their personal relationships as a result of this condition. In many areas there is a large imbalance between the need for diagnostic and treatment services and the resources available. This may be particularly true for adults with attention deficit disorder. We hope this book will contribute positively, in an educational sense, to those experiencing such difficulties.

Attention deficit disorder has been with us since ancient times. It is a relatively common problem affecting on the average, one child in every classroom in North America. The impact of this condition on children and families may be very significant. It commonly creates frustration, underachievement and conflict in many or all aspects of a child's life. Therefore it may be a cause of considerable unhappiness for both the child and the child's caregivers.

Some, but not all children, with attention deficit disorder are excessively active, a condition sometimes called hyperactivity. At one time this dramatic symptom was thought to occur in all children with attention deficit disorder and the term *hyperactivity* or *hyperactivity syndrome* became a commonly used title. In fact, over the past several decades a number of different names have been given to this entity as it has become better understood. Perhaps the most unnecessarily alarming name was an old one which considered the affected children to be brain damaged. Fortunately, the label *minimal brain damage*, was eventually replaced by a less unpleasant one, *minimal brain dysfunction*. Although it is true that some children with a clear-cut history of brain insult or damage manifest hyperactive and inattentive behavior, the vast majority of children suffering from attention deficit disorder have no history or other evidence of such insult or damage.

Since 1980 the scientific community has preferred the term *attention deficit disorder*, since it is now believed that the core symptom is an inherent weakness in the ability to concentrate – to sustain attention on relevant tasks and to maintain this attention until the task is completed. More recently, the term *attention deficit-hyperactivity disorder* has been proposed. However, there are still some investigators who believe that even this designation does not adequately describe the disorder, notwithstanding the fact that attentional difficulties are usually present in hyperactive children.

Throughout this book we use the terms *hyperactivity, attention deficit-hyperactivity disorder* (ADHD) and *attention deficit disorder* (ADD) interchangeably since all are currently in use and refer to the same condition. While currently we prefer the term attention deficit disorder, it is quite likely that as we gain more knowledge about the disorder we may yet give it a different name in the future. When possible, however, we have chosen to replace the word *hyperactivity* as a diagnostic term with the phrase *attention deficit disorder*, to emphasize the fundamental problem in this condition, namely a weakness of selective attention.Although attention deficit disorder is seen in individuals of all ages, we will confine our discussion to the disorder in children and adolescents. For this edition we have added a new chapter on attention deficit disorder in adolescence. Lastly, we have added new information on the possible causes of ADD based on more recent research.

The impetus for writing this book was provided by the parents and teachers of children attending our clinic, who requested a concise source of information on attention deficit disorder including the rationale for the recommended approaches to its treatment. Accordingly, this book is not intended to be a scientific discourse or the final word on attention deficit disorder. Rather, it is a short presentation of what is currently known and it should provide its readers with sufficient information to enable them to make informed treatment decisions.

Although controversial issues are discussed in the book, we do not provide specific references to scientific journals with respect to these issues. Instead, we provide the interested reader with a short list of additional readings which review these issues in more detail and are readily available at a local public or college library. Despite our attempt to refrain from using scientific jargon, occasionally we have found it necessary and therefore have italicized it within the text.

The authorship of this edition has been expanded to include Dr. Joel Fagan as a co-author and Carolyn Garbet-Smith MSW as a contributing author.

1   A Brief Historical Review

Our youth now loves luxury. They have bad manners, contempt for authority and disrespect for their elders. Children nowadays are tyrants.

– Socrates, 470 - 399 B.C.

The earliest known description of hyperactive behavior in a child was published in the 1845 children's storybook *Der Struwwelpeter (Unkempt Peter)*, by German physician Dr. Heinrich Hoffmann. The particular story of interest within this volume is "Die Geschichte vom Zappel Philipp." Some readers may be familiar with the entire translation which has been retained in its original doggerel verse. The first few lines are as follows:

> "Phil, stop acting like a worm
> The table is not a place to squirm.
> Thus speaks the father to this son,
> Severely says it, not in fun.
> Mother frowns and looks around
> Although she doesn't make a sound.
> But, Philipp will not take advice,
> He'll have his way at any price.
> He turns,
> And churns
> He wiggles
> And jiggles
> Here and there on the chair,
> Phil, these twists I cannot bear."

Toward the end of World War I many countries experienced an epidemic of brain infection (encephalitis), often associated with severe lethargy (sleep sickness or Von Economo's encephalitis lethargica). Many of the adults who survived the acute illness later developed a disorder known as Parkinson's syndrome which consists of muscle rigidity, an abnormal gait, shaky arms and hands, expressionless face, drooling, and disturbances of attention, memory, and emotion. On the other hand, some of the children who survived the acute illness developed a constellation of behavioral traits similar to what is now known as attention deficit disorder. This is the origin of the now discredited label *minimal brain damage*. However, it was soon realized that there were also many hyperactive children who had not suffered from encephalitis or any other cause of frank brain damage. Over the years the label was replaced by *minimal brain dysfunction*, which still lingers in both the scientific literature and popular writings.

In 1937 Dr. Charles A. Bradley, an American psychiatrist, described a group of institutionalized emotionally-disturbed children who responded to treatment with benzedrine, a stimulant drug. They showed increased interest in school work, better work habits and an improvement in their disruptive behavior. This improvement, which is contrary to intuition, could not be explained for many years. As will be seen later in this book, recent research on the functioning of the brain provides the promise of better understanding this mystery.

During the 1960s and early 1970s there was a wave of over-prescribing stimulant drugs for the treatment of many types of problem behaviors and failure at school. This overuse (far less common today) led to a justifiable outcry by many teachers, other professionals, parents, and even some physicians, against the practice of "medicating" children for their problem behaviors. These protests have led to a much more rational use of these medications and have provided an impetus to the vastly increased research into the causes and treatment of ADD. We are still not certain why stimulant drugs improve the behavior of only some children with attention deficit disorder and not others. Hundreds of scientists around the world are searching for answers to this and many other questions concerning this complex problem.

"Der Struwwelpeter (Unkempt Peter)

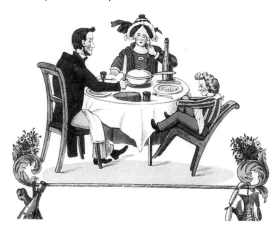

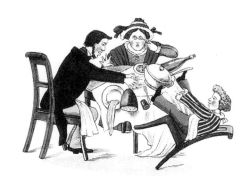

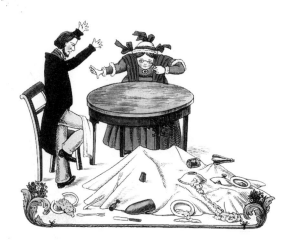

2   ADD - What is it?

*On every scientist's desk there is a drawer labelled "unknown"
in which he files what are at the moment unsolved questions,
lest through guesswork or impatient speculation he come upon
incorrect answers that will do him more harm than good. Man's
worst fault is opening the drawer too soon. His task is not to discover final answers but to win the best partial answers that he
can, from which others may move confidently against the unknown, to win better ones.*

– Homer W. Smith, 1895 - 1962

It is ironic that an abundance of writings on any topic,
whether in scientific journals or in popular magazines, is often
an indication of our inadequate understanding of that topic.
Consider a well-known condition such as poliomyelitis. Most
young readers of this book have not seen a child afflicted by
poliomyelitis but know that it is a disease which can be pre-
vented through routine immunization of children. Neither in
scientific journals nor in popular magazines does one find
articles about poliomyelitis. Now consider coronary heart disease and cancer, two common killers. It is hardly possible to
find a scientific journal or a popular magazine without an
article on these diseases. When we had learned a great deal
about poliomyelitis and its cause, we then learned how to
prevent it. It is no longer a major threat to our health and
therefore, people have little interest in reading or writing
about it. Not so with heart disease and cancer. We still have a
great deal to learn about them. As long as the search for their
cause and prevention goes on, scientists will publish the results of their investigations in professional journals. Attention
deficit disorder belongs to the same league. Between 1957 and
1960, less than three dozen articles appeared in the scientific
journals on the topic of hyperactivity. Twenty years later

(between 1977 and 1980) over seven thousand articles were published on this same subject. Between 1990 and 1994 over eight hundred additional articles were published, indicating a high level of ongoing concern. This continues to be the most researched childhood behavioral disorder and yet much remains to be learned about it. With each new piece of published research, it seems more questions remain to be answered. In this way scientific knowledge progresses.

Over the years this condition has been the source of both interest and controversy among psychiatrists, neurologists, pediatricians, psychologists, educators and the general public. Some reputable scientists have questioned its very existence. At times this controversy has even reached the political arena, when concerned citizens have requested lawmakers to ban certain forms of treatment.

Does hyperactivity really exist? To the distraught parent, or the harassed teacher, this is only an academic question. They know that it does. They experience it every day.

The hyperactive child, more often a boy than a girl, seems to be in constant and purposeless motion. He disrupts classroom activities and distracts other children. He talks loudly, excessively and out of turn. He interrupts others' conversation. When he does not talk, he often makes annoying noises. He seems to know the rules of appropriate behavior for his age but somehow is not capable of following these rules. Even when he is repeatedly scolded for inappropriate behavior, he seems to similarly misbehave over and over again. It is not that he is not motivated to comply with rules and social norms; he just seems to have a difficult time regulating his activities, emotions and thoughts. He often seems to daydream and not to listen even when he is spoken to directly. Although apparently looking at his mother or teacher during conversations, at times he seems to be looking right through them, preoccupied with distant thoughts.

He often changes his activities and seldom, if ever, completes tasks. His work is sloppy, careless and often incorrect. In family games he is a poor loser and attempts to change the game rules in order to win. The same tendency to change the rules leads to his being left out of group games whether in school or in the neighborhood. This type of behavior makes it difficult for him to find and/or keep friends even though he craves friendship. With adults he is often sassy. He is impulsive in style and acts without thinking. He will trip over objects and bump into doors and walls more often than expected. When given a new toy, his first impulse is to take it apart. When trying to reassemble it, he can become frustrated or distracted by other activities.

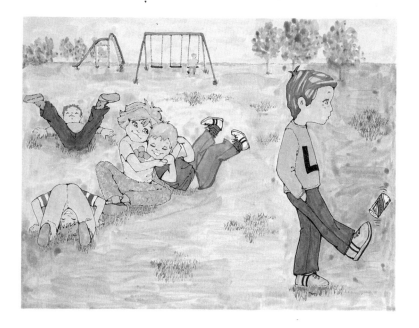

He may have difficulty falling asleep and occasionally his sleep is restless. If a preschooler, he may wake up frequently during the night to explore the household. He is an early riser and frequently is not in a good mood on waking up. Oddly enough, in one-on-one situations, such as in a doctor's office, he may behave perfectly normally. Occasionally he attempts to make that office look like a battle zone. He is often moody and has a low tolerance for frustration. As a result, he may show temper outbursts, with tendencies to bully and fight with other children. His school performance is often poor, or below expectation and he has low self-esteem.

The foregoing is representative of children with attention deficit disorder as a group. Fortunately, individual children seldom exhibit the complete array of abnormal behaviors described above. Even in the same child the intensity of abnormal behavior varies from time to time and from situation to situation. In fact the usual pattern is one of inconsistency.

Most of the behavioral problems common to these children result from inattention, impulsiveness and hyperactivity at a level which is inappropriate for their age. Naturally one has different expectations of a two-year-old toddler and a seven-year-old child in terms of attention span and behavior. It is also important to understand that many children who have the type of behavioral and learning problems described above are not physically hyperactive. For this reason, many professionals prefer to call the disorder *attention deficit disorder*; believing that the core problem of affected children is impaired attention rather than hyperactivity.

Their impaired attention makes it difficult for these children to focus and sustain their attention on a task and to avoid distraction. Impulsiveness makes it difficult for them to resist immediate temptations and modulate their behavior appropriately. When present, hyperactivity makes it difficult for them to regulate their activities so that they will be purposeful and goal-oriented.

Although some or all of the above described behaviors are frequently seen in these children, some professionals question whether we are sufficiently precise in our definition to be justified in calling the condition a distinct disorder by any name. They argue that terms such as hyperactivity and attention deficit disorder have resisted precise definition and cite some studies which have shown a relatively low level of agreement among parents, teachers and clinicians as to which children are hyperactive. While instruments for measurement of movements are available, there are no instruments which would precisely measure purposeless movements. When two different rating scales (usually questionnaires) are used to identify hyperactive children, parents and teachers do not always pick out the same children, even if both questionnaires have been validated and tested for reliability on the normal childhood population. Similarly, children who seem to be inattentive and easily distracted in the classroom can be seen totally absorbed in their favorite television shows. Is it then an *attention* deficit which is troublesome to these children or rather an *application* deficit? The phrase, "If Johnny could only apply himself" is familiar to many teachers and parents alike. Some clinicians argue that a seemingly inattentive child is capable of tuning in but is, in fact, not motivated to behave in accordance with the norms set for him by adults. He *chooses* not to apply himself. He may be considered to have an intention (application) deficit disorder. We do not agree with this interpretation of the problem.

Another point of disagreement among professional groups dealing with hyperactive-impulsive children has been the difficulty in distinguishing between attention deficit disorder and *conduct* disorders of childhood. In the past, some clinicians have believed that these are identical disorders. Most now argue that the two groups of disorders have many overlapping features, but that conduct disorders are characterized by the predominance of callous and remorseless antisocial behaviors, which violate the basic rights and property of others.

Some clinicians believe that there is little justification for coining a new name, such as attention deficit disorder, for what is not a distinct entity, since inattentiveness and restlessness are also seen commonly in association with a number of other conditions, notably learning disabilities. In response, other clinicians argue that there is a distinct difference between the restlessness and inattention of children with attention deficit disorder (ADD) and that of learning-disabled children: the learning disabled children, unlike ADD children, are not inattentive and restless outside the classroom and they were not so in their preschool years. Their restlessness and inattentiveness becomes apparent only when they are faced with academic challenges.

The major difficulty with learning-disabled children is their apparent inability to adequately process auditory and/or visual information which is presented to them while they are being taught to read, write and do arithmetic. Because of this difficulty in information-processing, learning-disabled children become restless and inattentive only in the classroom, or at home when they are expected to do homework. Their behavior in these situations could be compared to that of any of us who happen to be accidentally present in a scientific meeting of scholars, who are discussing topics beyond the limit of our understanding. In these situations, we too, may become restless and fidgety, with our minds wandering off to more meaningful thoughts. However, this daydreaming and restlessness would not persist when we left the scientific meeting.

What distinguishes the inattentiveness of children with attention deficit disorder from that of learning-disabled children is the range of settings in which this problem occurs. ADD children are apt to display abnormal behavior, with varying degrees of intensity, in all situations, including classroom, home, playground, supermarket, church and often in the physician's office. Furthermore, they may have displayed this behavior even in their preschool years. It must be reemphasized that even though this pattern of abnormal behavior may create conflict and underachievement in many or all settings, the severity of the problem may vary inconsistently from day to day. For many children this unpredictability is a hallmark of the disorder.

The inattentiveness of attention deficit disorder children is an intrinsic deficiency of their ability to focus their attention. It is a *primary* deficiency and is the principal cause of their learning problems. On the other hand, the inattentiveness of learning-disabled children is *secondary to*, (i.e., a result of) their information processing difficulties; unable to adequately succeed in learning tasks, their minds wander and they become daydreamers.

Inattention can also be the result of, or secondary to, other stressful factors such as depression and anxiety in the children, emotional disturbances in other family members, chaotic circumstances within the home, inappropriate expectations of the child by his parents or teachers and occasionally, a conscious effort on the part of the child not to pay attention in order to avoid humiliation (application deficit). There are, of course, children with mixed types of inattention. This classification of chronic inattention into primary and secondary types has therapeutic implications, in that only primary inattention and mixed primary and secondary types of inattention respond to medications. Secondary types of inattention require different types of intervention. The following table may serve to further clarify this useful distinction between various types of chronic inattention.

Finally it must be said that up to the present time, research has not made it clear whether attention deficit disorder is a single condition or a set of conditions. What is abundantly clear is that hyperactive and inattentive children are a complex and differing group of individuals who need our understanding.

A General Classification of Chronic Inattention in School-Age Children (modified from Levine, Melvine D. et al)

Subtypes	Description	Some Common Associations	Common Denominators
Primary attention deficit	Intrinsic inefficiencies of selective attention	Early onset of tempermental dysfunction Perinatal stress events Signs of neuromaturational delay Inattention in multiple settings and situations Sleep disorders	Purposeless selection of stimuli or activities Weak resistance to distraction
Secondary attention deficit	Inattention secondary to deficits in information processing	Visual perceptual motor problems Developmental language disabilities Deficits of sequential organization and short-term memory Signs of neuromaturational delay	Impersistence Inefficiencies of motor activity
	Inattention secondary to psychosocial, social and emotional disturbances	Family problems Emotional disturbance in other family members Primary depression and anxiety	Impulsiveness Academic underachievement or failure
	Apparent inattention resulting from inappropriate expectations, perceptions, or educational circumstances extrinsic to the child Inattention as a conscious strategy	Tendency toward inattention only in specific settings or situations Strong foci of interests and competence Discrepant perceptions of child by adults Task-specific attention weakness- "designed" to avoid humiliation	Social failure Performance inconsistency Diminished self-esteem
Mixed	Two or more subtypes	Relevant to subtypes	Insatiability

3   The Prevalence of ADD

Truth in all its kinds is most difficult to win; and truth in medi-cine is the most difficult of all.

— Peter mere Latham, 1789 - 1875

It should be clear from the foregoing discussion that it is difficult to talk about the prevalence of attention deficit disorder when there is incomplete agreement among scientists on what the disorder is. The American Psychiatric Association has attempted to devise diagnostic criteria for attention deficit disorder with or without hyperactivity in order to differentiate it from other disruptive behaviors of childhood. The first such attempt was made in 1981 in the third edition of the *Diagnostic and Statistical Manual*, or DSM III for short. This manual recognized three major types of attention deficit disorder: ADD with hyperactivity which consisted of inattention, impulsiveness and hyperactivity; ADD without hyperactivity; and ADD residual type, which described young adults (18 years of age and older) with a history of childhood ADD, with or without hyperactivity, whose signs and symptoms had persisted in varying degrees into adulthood. In 1987 and 1994 revised editions of this manual were published and included a revision of the diagnostic criteria for this disorder (see Chapter 5) which is now known as attention-deficit hyperactivity disorder (ADHD).

The published studies of the prevalence of attention deficit disorder have not always used the above diagnostic criteria. Nor is it always clear that when used, how strictly such criteria were applied in arriving at the diagnosis. It is not surprising then, that different prevalence rates have been found by different investigators. Furthermore, since hyperactivity, inattention and impulsiveness tend to change with maturity, different prevalence rates are obtained if a group of investigators study only kindergarten to Grade 4 students and others include children in junior high school as well.

Another confounding difficulty in establishing prevalence rates is the fact that many more boys suffer from this disorder than girls. If all children are pooled together a different prevalence rate is obtained than when only boys are studied. For example a study conducted in Italy reported that 20% of boys and 3% of girls were affected. However, the combined rate for all children, when boys and girls were pooled, was 12%.

Many prevalence studies use standardized questionnaires by which parents and teachers rate certain behaviors. Some questionnaires require the parent or teacher to respond whether a particular symptom, such as inattention, is present "sometimes, often, or always." Other questionnaires require the parent or teacher to respond whether the child displays a particular symptom "not at all, a little, pretty much, or very much." Thus using different techniques to establish the prevalence of this disorder will produce different results. Nonetheless, when similar techniques are used, there seems to be a general consensus among different studies reported from various countries. About 2 to 3% of girls and 6 to 9% of boys are reported to be affected in studies conducted in the United States, Great Britain, Australia, Germany and China. Somewhat higher prevalence rates are reported from Italy, Spain and New Zealand.

It is apparent that attention deficit disorder, whether or not accompanied by hyperactivity, is a common childhood behavior disorder. The question is how to diagnose and differentiate it from similar behavior disorders, which require different approaches to treatment. This will be discussed in Chapter 5. Before getting into the discussion of the diagnosis, we will briefly discuss the suspected causes of this challenging condition.

4   The Possible Causes

There are in fact two things, science and opinion; the former begets knowledge, the latter ignorance.

– Hippocrates, 460 - 400 B.C.

The most honest answer to the question "What causes ADD?" is, we do not know. Although theories abound, the cause of attention deficit disorder is still wrapped in mystery. There are many who believe that attention deficit disorder is a behavioral disorder with its cause rooted in the child's psychosocial environment. They argue that physicians, in collusion with drug companies and some teachers, have "medicalized" the disorder. There is no question that a chaotic home environment, marital discord, mental illness in the family, and many other stress-producing situations can cause behavioral problems in children. Neither is there any doubt that overcrowded classrooms, staffed by inadequately trained teachers, or boredom in a bright child (as well as a number of other psychosocial factors) can also be the cause of hyperactive behavior in some children. On the other hand, one must not hasten to blame psychosocial factors as the sole cause of the child's misbehavior. An extremely hyperactive child can create chaos both at home and in school, bring out the worst in the family and interfere with the teaching effectiveness of even the most capable teacher.

Based on our present knowledge, it appears that attention deficit hyperactivity disorder most likely has many causes and that in many hyperactive children varying degrees of psychosocial and biological factors may be operative at the same time. What follows is a brief description of *suspected* causes of ADD.

Brain Damage

The notion of a structural abnormality or brain damage as the cause of hyperactivity is still popular, particularly in non-scientific circles. Certainly, damage to the brain can cause behavioral changes consistent with the diagnosis of ADD. However, in the vast majority of children with ADD there is neither a history of prenatal injury to the fetus, nor of birth trauma, head injury or brain infection. However, when compared with non-ADD children, there is more frequently a history of maternal toxemia during pregnancy, complications of labor, or difficult births.

Head trauma is quite common in childhood, but it is nearly always impossible to relate it to the development of ADD associated behavior. A careful history may reveal that the child had some or all of the behavioral traits associated with ADD before the head injury. In fact, it is quite likely that the impulsive behavior of the hyperactive child may have led to his head trauma in the first place.

Repeated, careful and detailed neurological examinations of ADD children very seldom reveal signs of significant neurological abnormalities. The so-called minor or soft neurological signs such as poor gross or fine motor coordination skills that are often seen in some ADD children are difficult to interpret, since the same signs are also seen in many otherwise normal, non-ADD children. Electroencephalograms (EEG or brain wave recordings), brain scans and skull x-rays have never shown findings which would be diagnostically specific for ADD. It is doubtful that newer diagnostic tools such as magnetic resonance imaging (MRI) or positron emission tomography (PET) will be of value either in delineating the cause of ADD or diagnosing the disorder. What is certain is that with the increasing appearance in the popular press of articles about these technological advances, there will be a corresponding demand from some parents, encouraged by their neighbors, friends and some professionals that their children be given the benefit of investigation by these modern tools.

Biochemical Brain Malfunctions

Functional deficiencies of various parts of the brain have also been suspected of causing attention deficit disorder. The cause of these deficiencies is not known. Presently, there is a great deal of clinical and research evidence pointing to the important role of certain chemical substances produced by the brain, the so-called neurotransmitters, in the genesis of ADD. In particular an underproduction or an altered function of one of these neurotransmitters, dopamine, is believed to be possibly responsible for the behavioral traits of ADD children.

Genetic Influences

There is a significant body of evidence suggesting that genetic factors play a major role in the development of ADD. This evidence includes the following:

1. There is an increased incidence of reported histories of ADD amongst the parents and relatives of ADD children as compared to the parents and relatives of non-ADD children.

2. There is an increase in reported cases of ADD among the full siblings of ADD children as compared to their half siblings.

3. Many more boys than girls are affected by ADD which suggests a genetic predisposition in boys.

4. Studies on the occurrence of ADD in twins have demonstrated that when one of the twins has ADD, the likelihood of ADD in the other twin is greater if the twins are identical (monozygotic) than if they are non-identical (dizygotic).

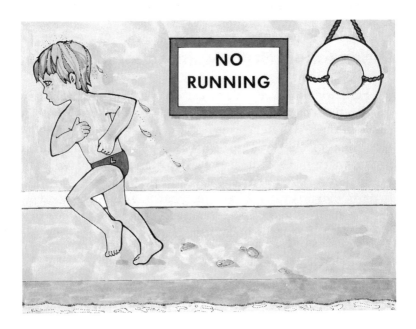

Infection

A recently published study provides interesting data which suggests that there may be a relationship between a common infection ("strepthroat") and the subsequent development of a number of childhood movement disorders such as hyperactivity or tics in some children. Further research in this field is necessary to confirm the findings of this thought-provoking study.

Maturational Lag

Since the behavior of hyperactive children is abnormal relative to their own age, but resembles the behavior of normal children of younger ages, it has been suggested that ADD children are slow in their development of certain functions of their brains. The problem with this assumption is that a lag suggests that eventually these children will "catch-up." Unfortunately some of the abnormal behavior of a significant number of hyperactive children persists, although less severely, into adulthood. Another problem with the notion of a lag is that it will encourage some professionals and parents to postpone effective treatment of the child, hoping that the child's brain will eventually mature. During the intervening period, however, the child and his family continue to suffer.

Poisons

Environmental poisons such as lead and other toxic metals have been implicated, but not proven, to cause ADD. It has been suggested that chronic exposure to lead or other toxic metals at concentrations too low to produce usual clinical signs of poisoning, may lead to subtle biochemical changes within the brain and to subsequent development of ADD symptoms in some children. Up to the present time we have no definitive evidence of such subtle poisonings.

Smoking and alcohol consumption during pregnancy have also been suspected as causes. We know that heavy alcohol consumption during pregnancy can lead to the development of Fetal Alcohol Syndrome. This syndrome consists of variable degrees of mental retardation, moderate growth deficiency, abnormal facial structures, weak attention, hyperactivity and a number of other abnormalities. We also know that babies born to smoking mothers are, on the whole, smaller than babies born to non-smokers. We do not know the possible subtle effects of minimal to moderate alcohol consumption or smoking on the developing fetus. As long as this is not known, it is prudent for pregnant women to refrain from drinking alcoholic beverages and smoking.

Hormone Abnormalities

Certain disturbances in the activity of the thyroid gland can cause ADD in rare circumstances. An overactivity of the thyroid gland (hyperthyroidism) may cause hyperactivity, weak attention and a fall in the rate of learning. However, this condition causes many other prominent symptoms which enable it to be recognized. It was recently reported that persons with an extremely rare, but different, abnormality in the functioning of thyroid hormone often have the symptoms of ADD. This condition is called "resistance to thyroid hormone" and is caused by an inability on the part of body cells to respond to thyroid hormones in the usual way. Although these thyroid abnormalities play no role in the overwhelming majority of children with ADD, they raise interesting and unanswered questions about the possible role of thyroid hormones upon the brain, particularly before birth.

It is not necessary to do thyroid testing on a child with ADD unless there are indications to do so in their history or physical examination.

Sensitivity to Fluorescent Light

Fluorescent light has been suggested as a possible cause of hyperactivity in some individuals. Carefully designed experiments have demonstrated conclusively that this is not true.

Food Sensitivity

The relationship between food and ADD is discussed in Chapter 10.

Summary

How all these possible causative factors might lead to the behavioral patterns observed in ADD children is not known. There are two theories which attempt to explain how this might take place. One postulates that the brains of ADD children are over-aroused; the other postulates their brains are under-aroused.

There is some laboratory evidence suggesting that dopamine deficiency leads to an under-arousal of the brain in ADD children, specifically under-arousal of those areas of the brain which create the ability to selectively focus attention on those stimuli most important for success, learning and pleasure. This ability is known as *selective attention*. Selective attention is the mental process which allows us to recognize and choose the central or most important stimulus from a complex, ever changing array of individual pieces of information, arriving at our brain on a moment-by-moment basis. This ability may be dependent upon the availability of appropriate levels of dopamine within certain areas of the brain. Attention deficit disorder is, indeed, a deficiency of selective attention.

Stimulant drugs increase the concentration of dopamine within these areas of the brain and this in turn is thought to result in an elevation of arousal and an increase in children's ability to focus their attention selectively. In this respect, stimulant drugs behave as they do in normal individuals and do not evoke a contradictory (paradoxical) response in ADD children.

It is interesting to note that Dr. C. Bradley, the originator of stimulant therapy in 1937, came to the same conclusion without knowing anything about dopamine or the under-arousal theory. He suggested that since certain parts of the brain have an inhibitory function over stimuli received by the brain through the peripheral nervous system, any stimulation of these parts would enhance their inhibitory function.

The following may help explain inhibitory function of the brain. At all times our brain receives, continuously and simultaneously, multiple stimuli through our senses. We hear sounds, see objects, smell odors and feel our clothing at the same time. However, our brain is programmed to *inhibit* and *ignore* irrelevant stimuli and concentrate on the important central stimulus. For example, while reading we may also hear people talk or feel the chair we are sitting on. Subconsciously, however, we ignore everything except the visual stimulus – the written words. This is the result of selective attention. This inhibition of irrelevant stimuli is an important part of our brain function. Without it we would be distracted by every sound, sight and smell, unable to concentrate on what we intend to do. Dr. Bradley suggested that this inhibitory function is impaired in hyperactive children and is restored by the action of stimulant drugs.

5   Diagnosis

Reason is immortal, all else mortal

            – Pythagoras, circa 582 - 500 B.C.

The ideal diagnostic evaluation of ADD would require the input of a team of professionals consisting of a specially trained physician, the child's teacher or a special education teacher, a psychologist, a social worker and possibly other professionals. Such teams are normally available only in certain hospital-based clinics. In the majority of cases, the parents must rely on the family physician to make a diagnosis in cooperation with the child's teacher.

Due to the fact that physicians have no precise way of measuring inattention, impulsiveness and hyperactivity, the diagnosis of attention deficit disorder remains a relatively difficult task for them. Purposeless over-activity in particular, is very difficult to measure objectively. A certain amount of activity is quite normal for a three-year-old. However, the same amount of activity is regarded as excessive for an eight-year-old. There are no standardized norms of activity, similar to those of height and weight, against which one can measure the child's activity level. A cynic once defined hyperactivity as the amount of activity which annoys the observer! Although there are some objective tests available for measuring impulsiveness and inattention, there are still some difficulties associated with their precise measurement and definition.

The difficulties associated with this lack of precise definition have hampered studies of attention deficit disorder for a considerable time. Researchers did not have a uniform and precise system of including children in, or excluding them from their studies. The diagnostic criteria introduced by the American Psychiatric Association in 1981 and revised in 1987 provided the scientists with an additional tool to help them with the clinical diagnosis of attention deficit disorder. Both 1981 and 1987 versions of the diagnostic criteria include guidelines for the exclusion of children with other disorders which may also be associated with hyperactivity or inattention. In 1994 these criteria were further revised in the fourth edition of the *American Psychiatric Association Diagnostic and Statistical Manual of Mental Disorders* (DSM-IV).

Diagnostic Criteria for Attention-Deficit Hyperactivity Disorder

Diagnostic and Statistical Manual of Mental Disorders, American Psychiatric Association, 1994 (DSM-IV).

A. Either **(1)** or **(2)**:

(1) Six (or more) of the following symptoms of *inattention* have persisted for at least 6 months, to a degree that is maladaptive and inconsistent with developmental level:

Inattention:

a. Often fails to give close attention to details or makes careless mistakes in schoolwork, work, or other activities

b. Often has difficulty sustaining attention in tasks or play activities

c. Often does not seem to listen when spoken to directly

d. Often does not follow through on instructions and fails to finish schoolwork, chores, or duties in the workplace (not due to oppositional behavior or failure to understand instructions)

e. Often has difficulty organizing tasks and activities

f. Often avoids, dislikes, or is reluctant to engage in tasks that require sustained mental effort (such as schoolwork or homework)

g. Often loses things necessary for tasks or activities (e.g., toys, school assignments, pencils, books, or tools)

h. Is often easily distracted by extraneous stimuli

i. Is often forgetful of daily activities

(2) Six (or more) of the following symptoms of *hyperactivity-impulsiveness* have persisted for at least 6 months to a degree that is maladaptive and inconsistent with developmental level:

Hyperactivity

a. Often fidgets with hands or feet, or squirms in seat

b. Often leaves seat in classroom or in other situations in which remaining seated is expected

c. Often runs about or climbs excessively in situations in which it is inappropriate (in adolescents or adults, may be limited to subjective feelings of restlessness)

d. Often has difficulty playing or engaging in leisure activities quietly

e. Is often "on the go" or often acts as if "driven by a motor"

f. Often talks excessively

Impulsiveness

g. Often blurts out answers before questions have been completed

h. Often has difficulty awaiting turn

i. Often interrupts or intrudes on others (e.g., butts into conversations or games)

B. Some hyperactive-impulsive or inattentive symptoms that caused impairment were present before 7 years.

C. Some impairment from the symptoms is present in two or more settings (e.g., at school, or work and at home).

D. There must be clear evidence of clinically significant impairment in social, academic, or occupational functioning.

E. The symptoms do not occur exclusively during the course of a Pervasive Developmental Disorder, Schizophrenia, or other psychotic disorders and are not better accounted for by another mental disorder (e.g., Mood Disorder, Anxiety Disorder, Dissociative Disorder, or a Personality Disorder)

Criteria for Severity of Attention-Deficit Hyperactivity Disorder

Mild: Few, if any, symptoms in excess of those required to make the diagnosis and only minimal or no impairment in school and social functioning.

Moderate: Symptoms or functional impairment intermediate between "mild" and "severe."

Severe: Many symptoms in excess of those required to make the diagnosis and significant pervasive impairment in functioning at home and school and with peers.

Although all versions of the diagnostic criteria still contain a great deal of subjectivity, they provide us with a standard format for taking a history of hyperactivity, inattention and impulsiveness. Everyone who has consulted a physician knows that an accurate history of an illness, along with a medical examination and laboratory investigations, constitute the essential elements of the diagnosis of that illness.

History

Since the behavior of ADD children varies from situation to situation (classroom versus physician's office) and from day to day in the same situation, it is important for the professionals to observe the child and to obtain behavioral reports from his parents and teachers. Inconsistency of behavior is a characteristic of ADD children. In the one-on-one situation of the physician's office such children often behave very normally.

The teachers and parents of the same children often report completely different behavior patterns. Experienced professionals rely heavily on these reports, since both teachers and parents have observed the child over a longer period of time and have had the opportunity to compare him with other children of the same age.

There are many standardized parent-teacher questionnaires for the purpose of obtaining information on child behavior. Perhaps the most well-known of these is the *Conners' Parent-Teacher questionnaire*. The abbreviated forms of this questionnaire are commonly used by many hospital-based clinics and physicians in private practice. Information obtained from the behavior-rating questionnaires is supplemented by the history of the child and is used to ascertain whether the child meets the diagnostic criteria developed by the American Psychiatric Association.

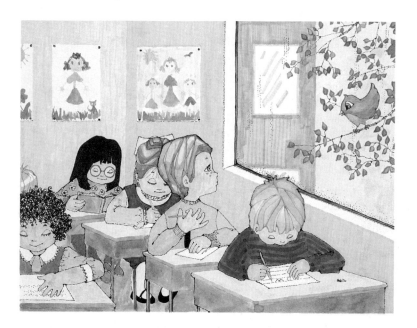

Parent Questionnaire

Instructions: Listed below are 14 items concerning children's behavior or the problems they sometimes have. Read each item carefully and decide how much you think this child has been displaying this behavior *today*.

Child's Name: _____

Parent's Name: _____

Today's Date: _____

Observation	Frequency (check one only)			
	Not at all	Just a little	Often	Almost always
1. Body in constant motion				
2. Difficulty sitting through a meal				
3. Constant squirming while watching TV or playing with toys				
4. Restless in car, church, while shopping, etc.				
5. Keeps changing activities or games				
6. Starts things without finishing them; does not complete tasks				
7. Difficulty playing cooperatively with others for more than a few minutes				
8. Does not seem to listen attentively or hear what you say				
9. Stares at things for long periods				
10. Talks too much or too loudly				

11. Interrupts or interferes with others' conversations or activities				
12. Mood changes quickly and unpredictably				
13. Easily frustrated; demands must be met immediately				
14. Acts without thinking				

Comments: _____

_____

_____

_____

_____

Teacher's Questionnaire

Instructions: Listed below are 13 items concerning
children's behavior or the problems they sometimes have.
Read each item carefully and decide how much you think
this child has been displaying this behavior *today*.

Child's Name: _____

Teacher's Name: _____

Today's Date: _____

Observation	*Frequency (check one only)*			
	Not at all	*Just a little*	*Often*	*Almost always*
1. Difficulty sitting still or excessive fidgeting, restlessness				
2. Difficulty staying seated, often on the go				
3. Starts things without finishing them; does not complete tasks				
4. Doesn't seem to listen attentively when spoken to				
5. Has difficulty following oral directions				
6. Easily distracted, difficulty concentrating				
7. Difficulty staying with a play activity				
8. Acts before thinking				
9. Has difficulty organizing work				
10. Needs a lot of supervision				

11. Interacts poorly with other children				
12. Demands must be met immediately, easily frustrated				
13. Mood changes quickly, cries, temper outbursts				

Comments: _____

_____

_____

_____

_____

It is important to realize that the process of diagnosis is not complete unless other disorders with similar patterns of behavior are ruled out. To do this, additional information must be obtained through a detailed interview of the parents. This usually includes the following:

- The onset, severity and frequency of the troublesome behaviors and their possible precipitating factors
- Any history of mental health problems or childhood hyperactivity in the parents and their siblings as well as in the child's siblings
- The number of children in the family and the amount and severity of sibling rivalry
- The presence of marital discord and other family stressors
- How the family is coping with the ADD child and what supports are available to them in the community
- The type and consistency of parental disciplinary measures and the child's response to them
- Maternal health problems during pregnancy and the events associated with labor, delivery and the early days of life
- Feeding and sleeping problems in the child during infancy
- Medications that the child may be taking

This type of careful and detailed history helps us to differentiate between ADD and other disruptive behavior disorders which have similar patterns of behavior, but require a different type of treatment. It also helps us to differentiate a child suffering from ADD from a learning-disabled child who has become frustrated with his inability to cope with the demands of school and has consequently developed fidgetiness, inattention and disruptive behavior. The learning-disabled child usually does not have a history of behavioral problems in preschool years, and his abnormal behavior is not apparent outside of school. It is important to re-emphasize that some

Check Out Receipt

Wapiti - Prince Albert - John M.
Cuelenaere
(306) 763-8496
http://www.jmcpl.ca/

Tuesday, March 22, 2016
5:07:07 PM
34712

Item: 33292002624033
Title: Attention deficit disorder :
a concise source of information
for parents and teachers
Material: Book
Due: 04/12/2016

Item: 33292011192089
Title: Epilepsy : information for
you and those who care about
you
Material: Book
Due: 04/12/2016

Item: 33292010997462
Title: Epilepsy explained : a
book for people who want to
know more
Material: Book
Due: 04/12/2016

Total items: 3

Thank You!

children may suffer from ADD, other behavioral disorders and a learning disorder at the same time. In such cases, each aspect of their problem must receive appropriate treatment. A learning-disabled child who is also suffering from ADD may require special education, stimulant medication therapy and, if necessary, behavior therapy. His family may also require supportive counselling.

Commonly Reported Behavior Patterns

As mentioned previously, the behavior of ADD children changes with age and maturity. Furthermore, ADD children do not always exhibit the full gamut of abnormal behavior which could possibly occur at their age. Appropriate treatment may modify their behaviors in a helpful way. What follows is a brief presentation of commonly *reported* behavior of ADD children. It is important to know that carefully designed research studies have demonstrated that some of these reported behaviors *do not*, in fact, occur more frequently in ADD children than they do in non-ADD children.

Infancy

In infancy, hyperactivity and irritability may be very noticeable features which may be present in the first year of life. The baby may be constantly wiggling and difficult to hold. Some mothers report excessive motor activity even before the child is born. In this stage of the child's development, his hyperactivity is not usually bothersome. His parents are usually more troubled by his disturbed pattern of feeding and sleeping. The child is often a poor feeder and is colicky. Usually colic is expected to disappear by three or four months of age. In children who are subsequently recognized to have ADD it may be present during the entire first year of life. During this time the child may demand almost constant attention by fussing and crying. He seems to need continuous entertainment. He may also have a difficult time falling asleep and may wake up frequently during the night. This may continue long beyond the age when most children begin to sleep through the night, that is, three to four months of age. After the child starts to crawl or walk, his hyperactivity and curiosity make him a first class explorer. This usually leads to more than his share of accidents through such activities as climbing up and falling from furniture and crawling under the kitchen sink to help himself to detergents, solvents, bleach or whatever else he can find. He seems to have several busy hands and is usually several steps ahead of his parents. Of course in this age group no one expects a baby to be entirely focussed and restrained. A great deal of acting without thinking is quite normal. What sets these children apart is their unusual difficulty in learning from past experience, which includes their parents' efforts to gradually shape their behavior.

Preschool Years

During the preschool years the excessive motor activity persists and may become even more prominent. Difficulties with attention and impulse control become more evident now. The child seems to go from activity to activity, and unless his parents or his play school teacher stand next to him, he will not remain with any activity for more than a very short period of time. He grabs toys from other children, disrupting their play and may show aggression towards them. He manages to become very unpopular with other children because he always wants to have his own way. He can learn the rules of good behavior, but somehow seems to be unable to follow these rules unless he is constantly reminded. Punishment of any sort does not seem to have any lasting effect on him. His impulsiveness continues, as does his tendency to be accident-prone. He may dash across the street without looking or get himself fearlessly into dangerous situations. Sleep difficulties may continue during this age. He may wake up in the middle of the night to raid the refrigerator, turn the television on or otherwise explore the household, wondering why everyone else is asleep. Some children are also early risers and often are not in a happy mood when they wake up. Mood swings and temper outbursts may become apparent at this age.

Early School Years

In the early years of school the most troublesome problem for the child is his poor ability to attend to learning tasks. Usually he has the ability to learn but he cannot attend long enough to do so. He starts tasks but leaves them incomplete because he is distracted by everything around him. Consequently he falls behind in his school work. However, if he is very bright he may learn quite well in spite of his poor ability to attend. Hyperactivity, in terms of excessive walking around the classroom, may or may not be present. More often than not, he is fidgety and constantly squirming. He talks loudly and out of turn and generally disrupts the class. He tends to answer the questions before the teacher has finished the sentence, that is if he is not daydreaming. His teacher reports that often he seems to be in a different world. He is disorganized and his work is usually quite messy. His disregard for rules continues and he is often left out of organized games. He may feel rejected and lonely; thus his self-esteem begins to suffer. His disturbed sleep pattern continues and he may now have nightmares or other signs of stress. His mood swings may also continue and his low level of tolerance for frustration will lead to impatience, increased temper outbursts and aggression towards his peers, parents and teacher.

Adolescence

After the child has reached ten or eleven years of age, his hyperactivity often becomes less noticeable, although he may still be fidgety and restless. During this period his poor impulse control severely interferes with his social relationships. His efforts at socialization may be awkward or insensitive to others' feelings. He may be craving friendship but becomes more isolated and in frustration may engage in antisocial behavior. His social and academic failure may lead to depression and further isolation.

Inattention and impulsiveness may continue into adulthood. The young adult may still be restless, although hyperactivity usually has disappeared. Underachievement, social awkwardness and frustration may be ongoing problems.

Medical Examination

Children of school age are often brought to the physician at the request of teachers. Not infrequently, the parents report that the child's teacher has recommended a medical examination for the child, including tests such as an electroencephalogram (brain wave recording). Occasionally the parents also ask for a brain scan or for some other expensive investigation.

It is the experience of all physicians who have worked with ADD and learning-disabled children that medical examination and routine blood and urine tests in these children almost invariably produce normal results. Likewise, detailed neurological examination of these children usually reveals no significant abnormalities.

Frequently one finds ADD children who show slight delays in the maturation of their nervous system have a poor ability to balance on one foot, hop or to move hands back and forth rapidly. They may also have difficulties knowing the right and left sides of their own body. These so-called "soft" neurological signs, however, are also seen in many children who have no attention or learning problems. Minor variations in electroencephalograms are seen in many ADD as well as normal children. Electroencephalograms are of no value in the diagnosis of ADD but they are most useful if there is any suggestion that the child may have a seizure problem. Promising new developments in the measurement of brain activity, through computer-assisted quantitative analysis of electroencephalograms, are now available. Some investigators claim that these techniques enable us to differentiate between learning and behavior disorders which are caused by brain dysfunction and those of environmental origin. The usefulness of the day-to-day clinical application of these techniques in the diagnosis of these disorders is still controversial.

It has, however, been reported that there may be subtle differences in the brain wave tracings of children with ADD, in comparison to children with normal selective attention. Furthermore, a number of investigators have claimed success in treating the symptoms of ADD using biofeedback techniques to modify brainwave patterns. This potentially useful treatment is still in the research stage and is not generally available.

Of course this does not mean that a medical examination is totally useless or unwarranted. The experienced physician knows that a good and complete medical examination, including an assessment of the child's hearing and vision, is essential for ruling out any possible physical problems, and assures the parents that the physician is thorough and interested in making sure that everything is done to come to a proper diagnosis. This, in turn, increases the parents' confidence and trust in their physician, and will lead to a better working relationship and adherence to recommended treatment. It should also reduce "doctor shopping," particularly where insured medical services are available and the parents do not have any out-of-pocket expenditures in seeking medical care. All told, there are no specific or definitive medical, neurological, or laboratory tests which can be used for making a reliable diagnosis of ADD. The patient's history provides us with the most useful diagnostic clues.

Psychological Tests

There are a number of psychological tests which may be very helpful in suggesting or confirming the diagnosis of ADD. Taken together with the history of the child's problem, these tests enable us to make a diagnosis of ADD with a relatively high degree of certainty.

The most commonly used test of intelligence in schools is the revised *Wechsler Intelligence Scales for Children* (WISC-R). This test has a number of sub-tests (arithmetic, coding, information and digit span) which require the child to focus and sustain his attention on test items. ADD children may score low in these sub-tests because of their characteristically low resistance to distraction. But at times, in the one-on-one (non-distracting) encounter with the psychologist the child may show strong attention, particularly if he understands the importance of the test and is highly motivated to succeed.

There are other tests which attempt to measure the child's selective and sustained attention. These include the *Paired Associate Learning Test* and the *Continuous Performance Test*. These tests of vigilance have been criticized for their inability to differentiate between a child who is not motivated (application deficit) and a child who is unable to focus his attention (attention deficit).

Another useful test is the *Matching Familiar Figures Test* (MFFT). The child is asked to look at a figure and then identify the same figure among a number of other similar, but slightly different, figures. The impulsive child often has a very short "latency period," that is, he quickly and without looking carefully points to a figure which may or may not be correct. He does not take time to think and compare; consequently he makes more mistakes than non-ADD children.

These and similar psychological tests are also available for preschool children. Interested teachers should consult their school psychologist for more information about psychological tests which may be useful in aiding the diagnosis of ADD.

Since many ADD children have associated academic difficulties, certain educational tests also provide very useful information, particularly in helping to differentiate between ADD children and those who are learning-disabled, and have become inattentive as a result of their inability to cope with their academic difficulties.

Hair Analysis

Occasionally parents ask for a hair analysis of their children to diagnose potential poisoning with lead or other toxic substances. Many commercial laboratories offer hair analysis services and often they give the results of their tests in impressive computer print-outs. Unfortunately, commercial hair analysis has not proven to be a reliable test for this purpose. A sample of a child's hair, divided in two parts, and sent simultaneously to the same commercial laboratory under two different fictitious names, produced two completely different results for one of us (Dr. Moghadam). Even if hair analysis were reliable and accurate, its results would not necessarily reflect the status of the tested elements in the child's brain or elsewhere in his body. Better tests for detecting environmental toxins in blood and urine are available to the child's physician, and can be ordered as indicated on the basis of the child's history and medical examination. Under most circumstances the need to consider this type of testing is extremely uncommon.

Allergy Tests

Some parents ask for allergy tests for their ADD children, believing that allergies play a role in ADD. However, no one has ever demonstrated a convincing cause-and-effect relationship between allergy and ADD, similar to those which exist between pollens and hayfever, or peanuts and hives. Therefore allergy testing, which may be costly and uncomfortable, has not been useful in this situation. There is some evidence that immunological disorders (including allergies) are seen more frequently in learning disabled and ADD children than in normal children. The relationship between food and hyperactivity is discussed in Chapter 10.

In summary, the diagnosis of ADD requires careful attention to the child's history which is obtained by interviewing the parents and whenever possible, the child himself. This information should be supplemented by behavior rating questionnaires completed by parents and teachers. This material together with the observation and examination of the child (and when appropriate the results of psychological and educational tests) can usually provide sufficient information for the accurate diagnosis of ADD. Unfortunately, there is no single, simple or more objective way to diagnose ADD with greater certainty.

6

Management: Drug Therapy

Healing is a matter of time, but it is also sometimes a matter of opportunity.

– Hippocrates, 460 - 400 B.C.

The aim of treatment of any disorder is either to cure it, or to improve the affected individual's sense of well-being. When the cause of a disorder is known, the treatment's aim is to eliminate it and to cure the disorder, whenever possible. However, when the cause of a disorder is not known, treatments are usually directed towards lessening the disturbing symptoms. Such is the case with the treatment of ADD. At present, there is no known cure for it. The aim of treatment is to improve the child's socialization skills and lessen conflict by enabling him to control his impulsive behavior and to better his school performance by improving the quality and span of his attention. This improvement in the child's socialization skills and school performance should then lead to an enhanced sense of self-esteem. An important by-product of the treatment is a reduction in the amount of purposeless movement and activity. Many ADD children improve as they get older and some even "outgrow" their problems. All, however, will suffer needlessly during their formative years if they are not given the benefit of presently available treatment.

In this chapter we will discuss the medical approaches to the treatment of ADD. The following chapters will deal with the equally important subject of behavior management of ADD children at home and in school. At the outset, it must be said that every treatment approach has its advocates. However, there is a substantial body of research evidence which indicates that presently, stimulant drugs are the most effective

Ideally a treatment program should include this medication, as well as behavior management advice, family counselling and a modified education program.

Stimulant Therapy

Stimulant drugs have been clearly shown to be a safe and effective treatment for the disabling symptoms of an attention deficit disorder. Although they do not cure the underlying problem, they often control its symptoms to a very important degree. They are the most effective means which exist to achieve this relief.

In spite of this, for many parents and teachers the idea of using medication in physically healthy children to help a behavior disorder is troublesome. The aim of this chapter is to provide useful information and reassurance.

Children with this disorder have a difficult time focussing and sustaining their attention on a task long enough to complete it. They are distracted by what they hear, see, feel, and even by their own thoughts. They are impulsive; they act before thinking and thus are unable to avoid disappointment and conflict. They need help to focus their attention and to pause and plan their actions. Stimulants enable them to do so. The goal of this treatment is not to drug children into submission or to convert them to "zombies." On the contrary, the goal of stimulant therapy is to give children control over their attention and behavior, and to enable them to think about the consequences of their behavior and act appropriately. These drugs help children to be attentive and successful, without suppressing their underlying alertness and personality. In essence, stimulants help these young people to liberate themselves from the imprisoning effects of "success deprivation" imposed by their disorder.

Many physicians prefer to combine the use of medication with a behavior management program for the child. Some physicians are reluctant to prescribe medication unless behavioral and educational modifications are instituted at the same time. This combined approach has been said to produce the best results. Since most family physicians and many pediatricians are neither qualified in developing a behavior management program, nor have sufficient time to make one, they must seek the assistance of other professionals. To be effective a behavior management program must be consistent at home and in school. This will be further discussed in the following chapters.

Since the aim of stimulant therapy is to improve the child's behavior and academic performance, the best results will be achieved through a coordinated effort of the child's physician, parents and teachers. Surpassing the teacher's role in helping to make the diagnosis are his or her observations of the child's response to treatment in the classroom, lunchroom and playground. The child's teacher is in an excellent position to observe if stimulant therapy is effective – more so than the prescribing physician. Periodic contacts between the child's physician and teacher make it possible for the physician to modify the child's treatment program based on his response during school hours.

Which children benefit from stimulant therapy?

The majority of ADD children, if properly diagnosed, will respond favorably to stimulant therapy. A few children, however, either do not respond at all, or show an adverse response. We have no means of knowing in advance how particular children may respond to stimulant drugs, since there are no specific predictive signs or symptoms. The child's history should provide the appropriately trained physician with sufficient information to allow a prediction of what child is *most likely* to respond favorably. If the child has had symptoms of ADD long before entering school, and his symptoms are present in varying degrees, in all situations, he is likely to benefit from stimulant therapy. As previously discussed, many children with ADD also suffer simultaneously from other conditions such as learning disabilities in specific subject areas. At the same time, others are victims of emotional distress caused by factors such as poorly functioning families.

These co-existing problems may lead the child's physician away from the diagnosis of ADD and the use of medications. The only way to know if a child will respond to stimulant therapy is to try it. When there is doubt about the underlying cause of inattention and distractibility it may be good practice to try stimulant therapy temporarily, so that no child who might benefit from it is overlooked. However, it is not good practice to prescribe medication without an adequate diagnosis and an appropriate plan to monitor the child's response to this treatment.

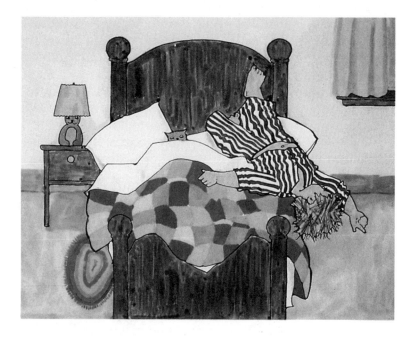

Drug Trials

Drug trials can also be used as a diagnostic tool, even though a favorable response to the medication does not necessarily confirm the diagnosis of ADD. This is because stimulant drugs tend to improve the attention span of normal individuals. Also many research studies have demonstrated the placebo effect of the drug therapy. The placebo effect is noted when the child's parents and/or teacher perceive an improvement in his behavior, even though he is not receiving a stimulant drug. For this reason many hospital-based clinics and some physicians in private practice resort to what is known as a blind trial of medication. In this type of trial, a pharmacist provides the child's parents with individually packed pills or capsules which may be either a stimulant drug or an inactive substance (a placebo). The pills or capsules look exactly the same. The pharmacist knows which day the child receives an active drug and which day a placebo; but the child, his physician, parents and teacher do not know this until the end of the trial. They are "blind" to this information.

There are a number of ways that drug trails can be carried out and each physician has his or her own preference. In all cases, the teachers and the parents are asked to complete either daily or weekly behavior rating questionnaires. If the child's behavior is improved significantly and consistently on medication days, as compared to placebo days, he is considered to be a favorable responder. Otherwise, the medication is discontinued or another medication is tried. A significant improvement is usually defined as at least a 20% improvement in behavior ratings of the child by his teacher and/or parents. Many physicians attach a greater significance to the teacher's ratings than to the parent's ratings because the child is normally with his teacher during the hours that the drug is most effective. If the drug trial continues during the weekend, the parents have a similar opportunity to observe the child's behavior during the peak hours of drug effectiveness. This will be discussed further in the following pages. Drug trials should rarely be attempted during the summer months when the teacher's input is not available.

Some physicians vary the dose of medication and placebo during the course of the trial in order to establish the most effective dosage for the child. Others use a fixed dose during the trial, and if the child responds favorably to stimulant therapy, they attempt to adjust the amount given following the trial.

Questions about Stimulant Drugs

What drugs are available for ADD treatment?

The most commonly used drug is *methylphenidate* which is better known by its brand name Ritalin. It is a relatively short-acting stimulant drug with some appetite suppressing properties. After taking it a change in the child's behavior is noticed within 20 to 30 minutes. The peak effectiveness lasts three to three and a half hours, and by four hours the effect of the medication has disappeared. Most of the drug is discharged from the child's body by that time. If the child receives his first dose in the morning he will usually require a second dose at noon in order to carry him through the school day. Older children may require a third dose late in the afternoon. Ritalin is also available in a sustained-release form; each dose is effective over a six to eight hour time span, thus eliminating the necessity of a noon-time dose. However, clinical experience shows that for some children the sustained-release form of Ritalin, because it may not be completely absorbed, is not as effective as the regular form, which is given in two or three doses throughout the day.

Methylphenidate is also available in a non-brand name (generic) form in some countries. Generic medications are usually less expensive than their brand name counterparts.

Another stimulant drug which is effective in treating ADD children is *dextroamphetamine,* available under its brand name, Dexedrine. It is in the family of drugs known as the *amphetamines.* It is very similar to *methylphenidate* in its action. It is available in tablets, each dose of which lasts four to six hours. It is also available in a slow-release capsule form which lasts for approximately 12 hours. This sustained period of action may be an important advantage for some children. For some it is a more potent appetite suppresser than Ritalin.

Another medication in this family is *pemoline* which is marketed under its brand name, Cylert. It is a long-acting stimulant drug which enables the child to take it only once each day. However, it may be somewhat difficult to adjust the dose of *pemoline* and for this reason it has not been as popular as *methylphenidate* with many physicians. Cylert's appetite suppressing properties may be less pronounced than Ritalin.

There are other (non-stimulant) medications which may be helpful for some children. Some physicians prescribe medications of the type known as tricyclic antidepressants. Examples of these include *imipramine* (brand name, Tofranil) and *desipramine* (brand names, Pertofrane and Norpramin). These drugs may succeed in strengthening concentration, particularly in children who are anxious and/or depressed. Some children who are not effectively helped by stimulants may be better helped by drugs of this type. However, these medications occasionally cause a number of potentially serious side effects which require careful explanation to parents and the need for laboratory tests to ensure their safe administration. As a result, the physicians who prescribe these drugs only do so when the stimulants have been ineffective when tried, or not well tolerated because of the side effects.

Other drugs which are used at times for ADD children are the *phenothiazines*, a family of medications known as neuroleptics or major tranquilizers. Examples include *thioridazine* (brand name, Mellaril) and *pericyazine* (brand name, Neuleptil). They are most often used as an aid to sleep for children who experience persistent and severe insomnia, either as a direct symptom of ADD or as a side effect of stimulant medication. As in the case of the tricyclic antidepressants these drugs may occasionally cause significant side effects. They should only be prescribed by physicians who have been trained to use them safely. Recently, it has been reported that the drug *clonidine* (brand name, Catapres) may be safely used to treat the insomnia that some children with ADD experience, either as a direct symptom, or a side effect of stimulant medication.

How safe are the drugs used in ADD treatment?

Methylphenidate and *dextroamphetamine* have been used for several decades and have proven remarkably safe and effective in their usual doses for the vast majority of children. There are rare individuals who experience adverse responses to these medications such as skin rashes or hives, much the same way some individuals respond to eating peanuts or shellfish. These are individual sensitivities and must be reported to the child's physician as soon as they are noted.

Although *pemoline* has been on the market also for quite a number of years, it has not been as widely studied as other stimulant drugs. It has adverse effects similar to other stimulant drugs in some children. A small number of children (1 to 2%) will experience a disturbance in liver function which usually causes no symptoms but is detectable through blood tests of liver function, which should be monitored for all children who take this drug.

There a number of medical reasons why stimulant drugs should not be used for certain children. These include cases of children with severe anxiety or depression, high blood pressure and chronic liver or kidney disease. A child with frequent seizures (convulsions) should not receive these drugs until their condition is treated effectively with appropriate anti-seizure (anticonvulsant) medication. The possible interactions between the stimulants and other drugs which the child may require should be studied before any stimulants are prescribed. The prescribing physician will be aware of these medical issues.

How do stimulant drugs work?

Some research studies suggest that stimulant drugs increase the amount of a neuro-transmitting chemical known as dopamine within the brain and in doing so, enable the child to gain control over his behavior, to pay attention to the most important stimulus entering his brain, to concentrate on the task at hand and to filter out irrelevant stimuli.

As mentioned previously, some clinicians believe that the core problem of ADD children may not be an attention deficit but an application deficit; that is, they consciously choose not to pay attention. Whether stimulant drugs improve the child's attention so that he can devote his mental resources to a task or improve his attitude so that he applies himself and does what he is capable of doing, is irrelevant. The fact is that stimulant drugs work in about 70% to 75% of ADD children. Their teachers and parents see an improvement in their attitude, behavior and work habits. The child becomes more available to instruction and thus easier to teach. These changes in the child seem to result from his increased ability to focus his attention.

When a child with ADD does not respond to the usual doses of stimulant drugs one should question the accuracy of the initial diagnosis and look for other causes to explain his behavior. These children may be good candidates for behavior therapy and their families may benefit from supportive counselling. Some children who respond adversely to a stimulant drug during the initial trial may respond favorably to smaller doses of the same drug or a different stimulant drug.

A number of years ago some investigators suggested that learning in ADD children improves only as long as they are taking stimulant drugs. It was feared that children would forget what they had learned when they discontinued taking their medication (state-dependent learning). Later research did not substantiate these concerns.

What is the best dose of stimulant drugs?

ADD children are a very diverse group of individuals and their response to medication varies considerably. On the whole, the younger the child, the smaller the dose required to achieve the desired effect. Normally, stimulant drugs are not prescribed for children under five or six years of age. The manufacturers of Ritalin and Cylert do not recommend their use for children under six years of age and the manufacturer of Dexedrine does not recommend its use for children under three years of age.

Some research studies indicate that the lower doses of stimulant drugs improve the child's attention span and the quality of his academic performance; somewhat higher doses improve his impulse control and consequently social interactions. The higher doses, according to these investigators, may have even a slightly deleterious effect on the child's academic performance. Other research studies contradict this finding and suggest the drugs have no differential effect on behavior and attention. The dose of stimulant drugs must be adjusted for each child, in order to obtain the most desirable overall response.

Many physicians start with a small dose based on the child's weight and increase the dose gradually, until, according to the child's teacher and parents, the best results are obtained. Other physicians start with a fixed average dose of one pill in the morning and one at noon, and obtain feedback from the child's teacher and parents in order to adjust the dose, if necessary. Some physicians find it more appropriate to discuss with the parents the rationale for stimulant therapy, the effects and side effects of the drug, and the signs and symptoms of an excessive dose. They then instruct the parents to increase or decrease the dose within certain limits (for example a maximum of four pills per day) until the best results are obtained. It is never wise for parents to give other than the recommended dose of medication without first consulting the physician who prescribed it.

As the child grows older the dose will usually have to be increased in order to maintain the same benefit. Some children with poor socialization skills may require a higher dose of stimulant medication after 10 or 11 years of age. Older children may need smaller doses as they mature.

When should the drug be taken?

Many physicians prefer that the drug be taken 10 to 15 minutes before breakfast and lunch. They believe that food in the child's stomach interferes with the absorption of the drug. Recent research casts doubt on this belief. Clinical experience suggests that for most children the effectiveness of the medication is not significantly effected by eating. Some children, however,seem to obtain a stronger benefit when the medicine is given before meals.

It is possible that in these cases the absorption of stimulant drugs is erratic when taken with meals. On some days the absorption may be rapid and on other days it may be prolonged. Taking the drug 10 to 15 minutes before meals may eliminate this erratic response pattern. For this reason, it is best for most parents to adhere to a program of giving the child's medication with a little water, 10 to 15 minutes before his meals unless there are reasons to the contrary.

Some older children may require a third dose of medication late in the afternoon if they have homework or other important evening activities, such as music lessons or organized sports. In such cases the child's appetite may be depressed during supper time. Should this happen, the child should be given a nutritious snack before bedtime in order to maintain his total daily nutritional intake.

How long should the drug be taken?

The simple answer to this question is, "As long as the child requires it." The best way to know whether the child continues to benefit from stimulant medications is to discontinue treatment periodically and observe the child's behavior. Many physicians recommend that the child be taken off medication for one to two weeks in the fall, usually several weeks after school has started. It is not a good idea to discontinue medication in the first weeks of the school year for two reasons. First, the beginning of the school year may be full of excitement for the child in a new classroom, with new classmates and a new teacher. Any change in the child's behavior may be due to this excitement rather than the discontinuation of his treatment. Second, if a true deterioration in the child's behavior follows the discontinuation of the treatment in the first days of school, he may be labelled as having a behavioral problem, a label which he may find difficult to shake off.

Temporary drug-free periods should also be avoided before important examinations and during the excitement of a holiday season or birthday party. The question of whether the teacher be informed at the point when medication is about to be discontinued, may be a difficult one. If the teacher is known to have strong feelings about the medication either in favor or against, it may be best not to do so in order to obtain an unbiased opinion about the child's learning and behavior while off the drug. On the other hand the teacher may be offended by this decision. In many cases there may be an important advantage in making the teacher aware of plans of this type so that the child may be appropriately observed in the classroom by the person who may be in the strongest position to know whether stimulant therapy should continue.

Many children learn strategies to focus and sustain their attention and to increase their impulse control during their adolescent years. They may no longer require medications at that point. Others continue to benefit from medication and should be encouraged to take it for as long as they need it. However, we know that many adolescents dislike taking prescribed drugs for a number of reasons. They may believe they no longer need them. Often they are embarrassed by having to take medication, fearing to appear different in the eyes of their peers and to be labelled. All adolescents are striving for independence, and many are stressed by their reliance on medication to achieve higher levels of attention and efficiency. Unfortunately, in many cases those who discontinue their medication are often those who benefit most from it.

There are also an increasing number of adults who continue taking stimulant drugs in order to maintain their powers of concentration, control their impulses and improve their success in social relationships and at their place of work.

Should stimulant drugs be taken continuously?

Many physicians believe that medication should be given only during school days. They recommend so-called "drug holidays," that is, discontinuing the drug on weekends, during school holidays and over the summer months. Other physicians believe that the child is learning in every situation, whether he be in school, at home, in church, on a playground, or in a mall, and needs to control his attention and impulses continuously in all situations. Thus, they recommend that the medication be given every day, much the same way as a diabetic child is given insulin every day. We believe that this decision should be made based the needs of the individual child. Some children function well outside of the classroom and do not require medication on weekends or school holidays. Many others experience significant problems in all settings and these children are helped by receiving medication every day. The ideal plan is for children to receive their medication in a flexible schedule which best meets their needs. For some children this means only on school days, while for others it means on weekends and holidays as well. For children who experience conflict and frustration during the evening or who have important homework assignments, it may be helpful to offer medication to cover these hours also.

If stimulant drugs help the child he should not be expected to take full responsibility for taking his own medication. Children and teenagers with ADD do not have sufficient memory and organizational skills to take their medicine reliably. Moreover, some young people are unenthused about taking medications of any sort and lack the conscious wish to take them regularly. In extreme cases they may even keep the pills in their mouth and spit them out whenever they are out of the sight of their parents and teachers. Many teenagers particularly dislike taking prescribed medications. However, if the medication has been effective in improving their school performance and social behavior, they should continue taking it. Achieving their confidence and cooperation may require a great deal of counselling by a trusted physician, parent or teacher. In the case of older children and adolescents these issues are best discussed openly, in a non-judgemental manner and often in private. The child's feelings should be respected. Both the benefits and the disadvantages of the medication should be acknowledged so that the child is supported in making a difficult decision.

What are the side effects of stimulant drugs?

Stimulant drugs are remarkably safe if they are given in appropriate doses; but they may have some short and long term side effects. The most common short term side effects are interference with the child's appetite and sleep. Stimulant drugs suppress appetite to some degree in many, but not all, children. Since they are short-acting, however, the child's appetite is normal in the vast majority of cases four to five hours after the drug is taken. In some children this is particularly true if the medication is taken 10 to 15 minutes before breakfast or lunch. If poor appetite persists regardless of when the drug is taken, either the medication dose should be adjusted or the child should be given a nutritious snack before bedtime, to compensate for his reduced food intake during the regular meal times. Very rarely a child's appetite remains poor even after a reduction in his drug dose. Bedtime snacks are most beneficial for these children. In some cases a different stimulant medication may be better tolerated.

Serious interference with sleep is usually not a problem when the child's last dose of daily medication is given at least four to five hours before bedtime, but it can be. If the child continues to have difficulty falling asleep, particularly if he is tired the next day, his medication dose should be reduced if possible and evening use of medication curtailed. Because of their long periods of action, the sustained release preparation of Dexedrine and Cylert may pose particular problems in this regard. When this occurs a change in medication or dosage form (i.e., changing from sustained release to regular acting) may be helpful. Rarely, when there is no alternative, the physician may consider adding a second medication for sleep.

There are a number of other, relatively uncommon, short term side effects of stimulant drugs. Most of these side effects are temporary – they disappear in a few days to a few weeks. Many of these so-called side effects have also been reported following treatment with placebos! It is not unusual for the young child to complain of abdominal pains or being sick in the stomach, and for the older child to experience a "butterfly feeling" in his stomach during the first few days of treatment. Younger children may complain of headaches and older children of light-headedness or dizziness.

Infrequently, a child on stimulant therapy becomes quiet or withdrawn and cries easily. This normally indicates that the dosage is excessive and a reduction in the dose will usually promptly eliminate this problem, while preserving the beneficial effects of the medication. It should be noted that some parents who have been accustomed to the child's hyperactivity, may interpret his reduced activity level following medication as an abnormal behavior. They may believe that their child has become emotionally depressed or unduly subdued, while in fact he has become normal. If the child truly does becomes subdued or lethargic, a reduction in the dose is usually indicated. Tremors, anxiety, irritability, over-talkativeness and dry mouth are signs of overdose. If a reduction in the dose does not eliminate these, the medication should be discontinued altogether.

Occasionally, the child's pulse rate and/or blood pressure increase slightly. Again, a reduction in the dose should bring these back to a normal level. The child's pulse rate, blood pressure, height and weight should be checked at least every six months while on medication.

In the early days of stimulant therapy, when these drugs were prescribed without the benefit of today's knowledge, their most common side effect was an interference with height and weight gain. This interference with the child's growth is very seldom a problem today, as long as the child's total nutrition intake remains adequate for growth. Some investigators have found changes in the concentration of growth hormone following stimulant therapy. However, most clinicians do not report an interference with growth and this speaks against any adverse effect of stimulant drugs on growth hormones. In our experience, few children's growth in height is slowed, even after several years of stimulant therapy. If this does occur, when medication is stopped, normal growth resumes immediatedly. More commonly, children may experience some slowing in weight gain due to the reduction in appetite brought on by the stimulants. Therefore, the child's weight should be carefully monitored by the physician, and if there is slowing, extra food should be offered during those hours in the day when the medication has worn off.

Psychological side effects of the drug may be either beneficial or harmful to the child. An improved sense of self-esteem is obviously a plus for the child. However, if the medication reinforces a child's belief that he has no control over his own behavior, that he has to take his pill in order to fight external forces which influence his behavior, he may develop a distorted view of his personal responsibility for his actions. This undesirable mindset may be reinforced by such remarks by the child's teacher, parents, siblings or peers such as, "Did you take your pill today?" or "Go and take your pill," whenever he shows a minor variation in behavior. It is the responsibility of physicians, parents and teachers to emphasize to the child that he is responsible for his own behavior, and that the pill only helps him in his efforts. In the same vein, any improvement in the child's behavior and interpersonal relationships should be credited to the child and not to the medication.

One of the beneficial side effects of stimulant drugs is a change in the parents' and teacher's attitude towards the child as a result of his improved behavior. Studies have shown that parents become less directive and less critical of their children following stimulant therapy. This positive change of attitude in adults toward the child can only be beneficial to the child's emotional well-being in the long run.

As a rule, stimulant medications should not be given to children with a personal or family history suggestive of Tourette's Syndrome. Tourette's Syndrome is characterized by multiple tics which may include complex patterns of movement involving the face, neck and, at times, the arms and legs. Affected individuals may make repeated noises (vocal tics) such as grunts, throat clearing, barks, coughs or use inappropriate words or obscenities. Many affected children also have an attention deficit disorder, which in itself may be very disabling. Treatment decisions in this setting may be quite complicated, since stimulant medications in some (but not all) children can accentuate their motor and vocal tics. When a child has both an attention deficit disorder and multiple tics a referral to an experienced and qualified consultant, such as a pediatric neurologist, is usually warranted.

Are stimulant drugs addictive?

Many years of experience have shown that children receiving stimulant drugs do not develop dependence on or tolerance to these drugs. On the contrary, as discussed earlier, many children would prefer not to take medication if they could avoid it. Stimulants improve selective attention without directly producing any pleasurable emotional changes which could potentially result in physical or psychological dependency. Certainly, many children who are mature enough to recognize the important benefits of this treatment are keen to continue with it. This is a reasonable choice and should not be confused with addiction to the drugs.

There are conflicting reports about increased risk of alcohol or other substance abuse among adolescents and adults who were hyperactive in childhood as compared with the general adolescent and adult population. This increased risk appears to be true, primarily for a subgroup of hyperactive children who are also aggressive, come from poor socio-economic backgrounds or chaotic home environments, are of lower intelligence and continue to have poor self-esteem. It should be noted that the increased risk, if any, has been determined from the studies of *groups* of ADD children. There are no predictive signs which would indicate a poor prognosis for an *individual* child with ADD. Indeed, it appears very likely that the medication-induced improvement in the child's behavior and self-esteem will decrease his risk of alcohol and drug abuse in later years. At present, no clear-cut correlation has been established between the use of stimulant drugs for the treatment of ADD, and the future abuse rate (increased or decreased) of alcohol and illegal street drugs by these children. This is further discussed in Chapter 12.

Are stimulant drugs used for preschool children?

Attention deficit disorder, unless associated with extreme hyperactivity and impulsiveness, is seldom diagnosed in preschool children. When diagnosed, most physicians prefer not to use stimulant drugs in this age group. Unlike their school years, when children are expected to conform to the rules of the classroom, it is felt that, during the preschool stage of the child's development, their behavior can be modified with behavior management programs designed to be used by their parents. As stated earlier, most family physicians and many pediatricians have little training in this field. They will be most helpful to the families if they refer these children to child psychiatrists, child psychologists, qualified social workers or, if available, specialized clinics in their communities.

Most parents of hyperactive preschool children are tolerant of their behaviors. However, some very difficult children disrupt the family life to such an extent that medical intervention may become necessary. These are highly inattentive and impulsive children whose behavior is impossible to manage effectively, and whose safety may be at risk because of their poor judgement and the exasperation they produce in their caregivers. In such cases, small doses of stimulant drugs are occasionally prescribed by some physicians.

Other drugs

Sedatives such as *phenobarbital* are usually ineffective in the treatment of hyperactive preschool children. Tranquilizers such as *valium* or antidepressants such as *tofranil* are not recommended for the treatment of preschool children since they have not been shown to be safe for prolonged use in this age group. There is probably one exception to this general rule. When the parents cannot find a willing babysitter for the child and must take the child to a special occasion such as a church wedding, a small dose of tranquilizer may be prescribed for the child. Some may argue that in these situations the parents benefit more from the tranquilizer than does the child, as the following anecdote may demonstrate: In the early days of tranquilizers, a distraught mother asked her physician once again for advice regarding her hyperactive four-year-old son. On previous occasions, she had found her physician's advice neither useful nor practical. This time the physician told her that there was a new drug on the market which might help. The desperate mother accepted the prescription and left the office. When she returned a month later for a follow-up visit, her physician immediately inquired about Johnny, to which she responded with a shrug and a smile, "Who cares?"

There are a number of other drugs which are prescribed for the treatment of ADD primarily by psychiatrists or used by researchers searching for more effective means of treatment. For the sake of brevity these drugs are not discussed here. Stimulant drugs are by far the most commonly prescribed medications for the treatment of ADD.

In this chapter, we have discussed the medical treatment of ADD children at some length. It has not been our intention to present stimulant drugs as a panacea. There is no question about the short-term beneficial effects of stimulant drugs. If the ADD child can also be taught to gain better control over his own behavior through non-medicinal means, it would be unreasonable to deny him and his family the benefits of such treatment. Indeed, due to the complexity of ADD and the wide range of problems experienced by ADD children, it is best to offer the child and his family a variety of treatment approaches. Other forms of non-drug management will be discussed in the following chapters.

7   Behavior Management

From the moment of his birth the customs into which an individual is born shape his experience and behavior. By the time he can talk he is the little creature of his culture.

— Ruth Fulton Benedict, 1887-1948

M. Haug

Over the years many forms of psychological treatment have been tried with ADD children, but only a few have proven to be of significant benefit for the majority. These fall broadly under the categories of *behavior modification* (also known as *behavior therapy*) and *cognitive behavioral therapy*. These strategies are also discussed in Chapter 9.

Behavior Modification

For some people behavior modification has distasteful connotations. They equate it with brain-washing, imposing our will on children, bribing, psychological torture and forcing children into submission. All of these are repugnant and far from the truth. Behavior modification is based on the principle that our behavior is influenced and can be changed by the type of response it produces.

The behavior of a newborn infant is governed primarily by the basic internal drives of hunger, discomfort, pain, etc. As the infant grows, his behavior is increasingly influenced by the behavior and responses of his parents and other people. In adult life societal norms and rules become major factors governing his behavior. Behavior modification draws upon these basic facts and attempts to bring about a change in the child's behavior by modifying the behavioral responses of parents, teachers and others around him. What follows is a very brief description of the aims and the principles of behavior modification.

Aims

Although behavior modification programs are devised by psychologists or psychiatrists, the programs are normally carried out by parents and teachers. The professionals teach the principles and procedures of behavior modification to parents and teachers of ADD children to assist them in their efforts to bring the child's behavior more into line with societal norms and expectations. The goal is to teach the child how to behave properly, to recognize and follow rules, to cooperate with others, to be a better listener, etc. It is anticipated that when the child learns these skills, he will have more positive and rewarding relationships with other people and will function more productively in the home, school and community.

Principles

Behavior modification is based on the observation that the behavior of a person is governed to a large extent by the consequences that follow the performance of that behavior. If an action is followed by a pleasant or rewarding response, that action is more likely to be repeated by the person in similar circumstances in the future; this behavior is said to have been "reinforced." On the other hand, if the action is followed by an unpleasant or punishing experience, the action is less likely to recur. By applying this basic law of psychology we are able to influence one another's behavior. We cannot escape influencing others or avoid being influenced by others. In the past several decades much study has been devoted to understanding how we influence one another and also what the most effective ways of exerting these influences are. We have learned that we can consciously and purposefully choose ways of interacting with others which will have a greater likelihood of obtaining the behavioral effects desired.

Behavior modification makes use of this principle and teaches parents and teachers to more systematically acknowledge and reward the good things the ADD child does (e.g., cooperates, pays attention, sits still, plays quietly and completes a task) and to avoid reinforcing his undesirable behaviors. Minor undesirable behaviors are best ignored. It comes as a surprise to many people that nagging, criticizing and even spanking may actually reinforce the very behavior they are hoping to eliminate! This is because there are all kinds of *attention* and children find attention being paid to them rewarding, even the *negative* kinds of attention. It is generally more punishing to a child to be ignored than to be reprimanded.

If an undesirable behavior can be consistently ignored by everyone in the child's environment, often it will eventually be eliminated, or at least be reduced, to occurring infrequently. If ignoring is ineffective or impractical (as in the case of major infractions of rules of good behavior or potentially dangerous behavior) a procedure called "response-cost" is an effective alternative. In this procedure the child is given "points" for avoiding undesirable behavior. Earned "points" can be exchanged for various rewards. Alternatively, the child may be given a set number of points at the outset. However, he *loses* a portion of these points every time he displays the undesirable behavior – he suffers a response-cost.

It is important to recognize that the child may never have learned how to perform the desired behaviors or how to perform them well. One can shape the performance of a desired behavior over time by rewarding first, the child's effort, then the noted improvements and finally, the correctly performed behavior.

Use of Behavior Modification

The same principles apply to the management of the ADD child's behavior as to that of any other child. However, due to the nature of this disorder, a number of modifications to the general rules are advisable.

1. ADD children are at the mercy of their impulses. They are not always masters of their own fate. They also have a short attention span and fleeting interests. For these reasons it is necessary to give the child particularly clear and explicit messages about the behaviors of concern, ensuring that his attention has been drawn to the matter, and that he understands the nature of his inappropriate behavior and the purpose of correcting it.

2. It is necessary to deliver reinforcements and response-costs promptly and consistently, so that the child is more likely to note the connection between the behavior and its consequences.

3. Since ADD children tend to become bored very quickly and easily, one cannot use the same reinforcer for a behavior repeatedly without running the risk of it losing its effectiveness. One must use a variety of reinforcers to maintain the child's interest and motivation to perform.

4. Finally, it is helpful to remember that with this group of children it is usually better to work on changing one undesirable behavior at a time.

Summary

Behavior modification is largely a matter of common sense. However, while simple to explain, it is often difficult to put into practice, particularly when there is a long history of unhappy and unsuccessful interaction between parents and the child. Professional help can be invaluable in helping families to break out of such a pattern and to learn new and more positive ways of influencing one another. It is the most effective tool we currently have in treating the pre-school age child for whom stimulant medication is often not prescribed. It is also a significant supplement for an older child, even one who is responding favorably to stimulant medication, as it maximizes the child's opportunities for learning, achieving social success and developing positive self-esteem.

It is important for parents and teachers to know that the responsibility for changing a child's behavior is theirs; psychologists and psychiatrists can only advise. In addition, parents must know that their involvement in the treatment program is normally in terms of years, rather than weeks or months.

For readers interested in learning more about behavior management, Wesley Becker's book *Parents are Teachers* is highly recommended (see Suggested Readings, p. 128)

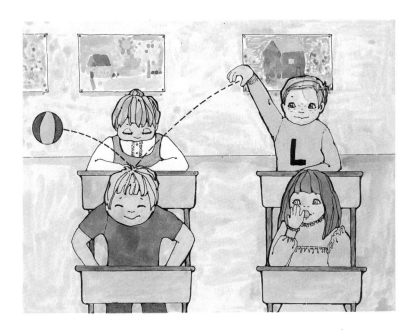

Limitations of Behavior Therapy

While behavior modification methods are very helpful in improving a child's behavior, in most cases they do not constitute a complete "cure." Their major limitation lies in the fact that the child's behavior remains to a large extent under *exter-*

nal control – that of parents, teachers, et al., rather than within the child himself. The obvious drawback to this is that the child will not always be in the presence of these helpers, and particularly as he gets older, he will be called upon more and more to exert self-control.

Other limitations to behavior therapy include the following:

1. The undesirable behavior may recur following the conclusion of behavior therapy. If the old pre-treatment reinforcement patterns are resumed, the child's behavior will likely revert back into the old undesirable patterns as well.

2. For a variety of reasons some ADD children do not respond to behavior therapy. Among the more important factors are:

    a) unless the methods are used very consistently by all persons who interact regularly with the child, their effectiveness is limited.

    b) a child who is a positive responder to medication may become unresponsive to behavior therapy when his medication is discontinued.

    c) if there are serious emotional or interpersonal relationship problems in the family, behavior therapy is unlikely to be successful until these have been addressed.

3. Experience has shown that behavior therapy often is ineffective for children of single parents. Because there are so many competing demands on their time, energy and attention, it is difficult for single parents to apply the procedures with the consistency required in order for them to be effective.

4. It is important for teachers to cooperate with behavior therapy. However, many teachers are unable to carry out a program of behavior modification due to the demands and responsibilities of teaching a large classroom. As is the case with parents, without teachers'

commitment to the behavior modification program, it will not achieve its fullest potential.

5. Finally it must be said that evidence for long term effectiveness of behavior modification is still lacking.

Acquisition of Self-Control

In the course of normal development children acquire increasingly sophisticated language skills. They also learn what is known as "inner speech," the ability to form in one's mind a linguistic representation of objects, events, experiences and relationships.We all engage in an internal dialogue within ourselves when we think and plan our actions. This internal conversation that we carry on in our minds plays an essential role in shaping our behavior. We can remind ourselves verbally of the consequences of our actions; we can in a sense bring the future symbolically into the present and let it influence our behavior in the here-and-now. Likewise, we can remind ourselves of our past actions and their consequences and use this information to predict the results of various behavioral options and thus choose our behavior accordingly. We can also benefit from the accumulated experiences of other people distilled into the form of social norms and rules.

However, ADD children seem to have difficulty in developing effective control over their behavior through the use of their inner speech. Often, unable to inhibit their responses to the more immediately available gratifications, they ignore the more distant, but ultimately more satisfying ones. The may "know" the rules. They may have the best of intentions. But they lack the self-control necessary to persist in the pursuit of a long range goal in the face of difficulties or distractions. The poor use of this inner speech also results in their having poor problem-solving skills. Instead of becoming more reflective and able to implement plans when "the going gets tough" they tend to become even more hasty, impulsive and random in their efforts. They do not "talk themselves through" a problem.

Cognitive Behavior Therapy

Aims

As applied to impulsive children (including those with ADD), cognitive behavior therapy aims to improve their problem-solving skills and self-control by teaching them to use "inner speech" to guide their behavior. They are taught to *monitor* and *evaluate* their own performances, to *instruct* themselves to follow a sequence of steps in problem-solving and to provide themselves with appropriate, constructive *consequences* for their own behavior. It is most effective when used with older children (i.e., eight years of age and older), as they are more likely to have the necessary mental maturity to grasp the procedure.

Procedures

Through a combination of discussion, demonstration (done by the therapist) and rehearsal, the child is taught a set of verbal self-instructions along the following lines :

Step 1 – problem definition:

"Stop! What is the problem?"
"What am I supposed to do?"

Step 2 – problem approach:

"I need to make a plan."
"What are some plans?"
"I have to look at all possibilities."
"What are my choices?"

Step 3 – focusing of attention:

"I need to concentrate."
(This step may be placed either earlier or later in the sequence, depending on the needs of the child.)

Step 4 – choosing a response:

"What is the best plan?"
"I think this is the answer."

Step 5 – carrying out the response:

"Carry out the plan."

Step 6 – self-evaluation:

"Did the plan work?"
"Did I do it right?"

Step 7 – self-reinforcement or coping statement:

"Great! I did a good job!" or "Oh, I made a mistake. Next time I'll go slower and concentrate harder and maybe I will get it right."

The wording, sequence and number of steps are tailored to the needs and abilities of the individual child. They are altered as necessary to fit specific problems. The child practices using the steps, first on impersonal and non-threatening problems such as games, maze puzzles, and school-like tasks (i.e., simple arithmetic problems) and then on more emotionally difficult interpersonal problems. Hypothetical problems are role-played by the therapist and child (or a group of children) using the verbal self-instructions to generate more socially appropriate responses. Practice within the therapy sessions is supplemented by "homework" assignments requiring the child to apply these steps to problems encountered at home and at school. Parents and teachers are also taught how to prompt the child to use the steps if he forgets to use them in a situation where they might be helpful.

Like behavior modification, cognitive behavior therapy seems to be an effective tool for improving the behavior of children with ADD. However, its long term effectiveness has not been established as yet.

Social Skills Training

General self-control training must often be supplemented with specific training in observational skills (recognition of other's feelings, non-verbal social cues, etc.), perspective-taking (putting one's self in another's shoes), conversation and play skills, relaxation and other areas. The social skill deficits that so often accompany ADD are frequently the most trouble-some aspects of this disorder. Because of their attention deficit, these children may fail to acquire an awareness and under-standing of the subtleties of social interactions; and because of their poor impulse control, they may say and do things that alienate others, often regretting it afterwards, but not profiting from the experience. They may have difficulty in making or in keeping friends or both. Chronic social failure is likely to lead to demoralization and lowered self-esteem and the further problems that these create. Thus, it is of vital importance that these children be given direct instructions in the social skills they lack, as it cannot be assumed that they will just "pick them up" the way most children do. Parents and other caring adults should take pains to provide opportunities for social success (e.g., through physical education) and should assist the child in learning to solve his problems. They should seek the help of mental health professionals to supplement their efforts when necessary.

8 Parental and Family Issues

In adversity remember to keep an even mind.

— Horace, 65 - 8 B.C.

C. McFee

In previous chapters we have discussed the behavioral patterns of children with ADD and the various forms of treatment. We have focussed primarily on the needs of the child. In this chapter we will discuss the impact of this condition on the family and how the family may be helped to cope with the challenges they may experience in having a child with ADD.

Common Concerns and Problems

Raising a child with ADD may be a formidable challenge. Many parents of affected children suspect from an early age that their child is different from others in behavior and response to discipline. Despite these concerns it may take some time before the correct diagnosis is made. In their discussions with professionals parents may feel that their concerns are down-played. Relatives, friends and neighbors often suggest that the child's annoying conduct is due to poor child-rearing practices. It is not surprising that many parents come away from these encounters feeling guilty and insecure. These parents, like all other parents, have hopes and dreams for their children and clear ideas of how their relationship with their children should be. Over time a number of unhappy emotions may blot out their original optimism. Many experience a sense of failure when their best efforts seem insufficient. Over time they may come to resent the child for monopolizing their time and energy. The child becomes identified as the "difficult one" in the family, the one who is expected to misbehave. Consequently, they may feel relieved when the correct diagnosis is made.

Self-Esteem Issues

Parents who have been successful in raising other children become frustrated when they realize that their parenting skills are comparatively ineffective with the ADD child, particularly when the usual praise, rewards and punishments do not work. They find it difficult to modify their expectations of the ADD child while maintaining fairness for other children. Their inability to teach their child to succeed and to effectively reduce conflict within the family create feelings of inadequacy as well as fears for the future. For these reasons it is essential for parents to discover and practice ways to strengthen their own positive self-worth.

The child's anger and frustration are also a major concern for the parents. The ADD child often does not see the connection between his behavior and the reactions of others. His unusual and annoying behavior leads to rejection by peers and resentment by siblings. Other children may "pick on him" for reasons that he cannot understand. If, in addition to struggling socially, the child is also doing badly at school, his self esteem will all but disappear. It is no wonder that at times, parents may feel overwhelmed when faced with these difficulties. Often, an ongoing challenge for parents is to help their child find social and recreational situations in which he can succeed.

The Effects of the ADD Child on the Family

The extraordinary expenditure of time and energy required in parenting an ADD child (often with few or no measurable results) imposes stress in marital relationships and undermines family harmony. Parents may disagree on how the child is to be understood and disciplined. One parent may view the other as overly harsh or forgiving. Both parents experience the child's unhappiness deeply but in their own way. These differences may give rise to conflict and confusion which may adversely effect the very best parenting intentions. Differences in expectations and responses between parents add to the child's insecurity. All of this can have a significant negative impact on the marital relationship.

In addition to working through and resolving these differences, parents often need to respond to the siblings' reactions and their stresses. Siblings of an ADD child often feel neglected due to the attention focused on the ADD child and resent the different behavioral expectations within the family. They often feel that the ADD child is the instigator of conflicts and blame him unfailingly. The parents, caught in this dilemma, find it difficult to respond rationally in resolving these conflicts. Over time their growing sense of helplessness and frustration can evolve into resentment toward the ADD child, which may increase the risk of losing control, and physically or emotionally harming the child. When families are troubled by other personal and marital problems, the added stress caused by the behavior of an ADD child may make it even more difficult for couples to cope. This combination of circumstances may eventually lead to family breakdown.

There are great challenges for all parents trying to find methods of coping with the stresses of ADD children. For single parents the stress and other unhappy emotions which occur in parenting an ADD child may be more profound and potentially exhausting.

Most parents have had little experience in observing the wide differences which occur in the behavior and development of normal children. Lack of experience makes it difficult for them to place their child's ADD problems in a comfortable context. This is particularly true for those parents whose first, and perhaps only child, has ADD.

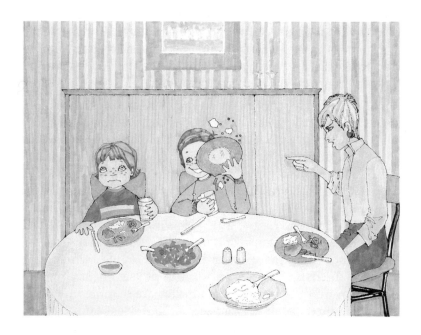

The Effects of External Forces on the Family

Parents of ADD children often have troubled relationships with others outside their immediate family. Extended families (grandparents, uncles, aunts, etc.), friends, neighbors, teachers, and other professionals, often present parents with unsolicited, conflicting and confusing advice on how they should raise their children. The search for a diagnosis may take years and involve parents in meeting with a series of professionals who may be uninformed and/or unhelpful. They come away from these episodes feeling angry and defensive, believing that they are being held responsible for their child's misbehavior. They perceive subtle or sometimes direct messages implying marital problems or poor parenting skills. They hear that they have inappropriate expectations of their children or are not sufficiently consistent in dealing with bad behavior. They may feel blamed for not following through with recommendations for treatment, or for lacking love and affection for their children. These painful encounters contribute to feelings of inadequacy and failure, which may then lead to an increased sense of isolation, as well as a defensive and sometimes even hostile attitude towards professionals. They begin to view the professionals as recommending treatments which arise from an assumption that they are inadequate parents.

Parents' Reactions to the Diagnosis

Often parents have consulted a number of physicians (or other professionals) regarding their child's difficult behavior before ADD is finally diagnosed. Frequently there is a two or three year lapse from the time parents suspect that there is something wrong with their child until the diagnosis is made.

Parents' reactions vary when at last the diagnosis is explained to them. Some feel relieved that they are no longer seen as the cause of their child's problems. Others feel pressured or overwhelmed by the large amount of information presented to them. Almost all parents struggle with numerous emotions at this time. Even when the diagnosis is thoroughly explained to them, they will wonder whether their child really has little control over his behavior or if he is just uncooperative and stubborn. They may still question whether he can hear them well or if, as the doctor explained, his listening (attentional) skills are impaired. They are concerned about his education and future success as an adult. They worry that he may become delinquent and eventually end up in prison. They struggle with the difficult decision as to whether or not they should put him on medication. Other related questions and concerns regarding the cause, the diagnosis, treatment and outcome are in their minds. Many parents go home and talk with relatives, friends and neighbors. They often become more confused when they hear scepticism about the diagnosis and frightening stories about the drugs. Mothers are usually more accepting of this diagnosis than fathers, as they are traditionally more directly involved with the child in attending appointments with the physician, teacher, or other professionals. If both parents receive comparable information about ADD at the outset, then in time, both should come to a similar level of acceptance.

Parents need an opportunity to deal with their mixed emotions. They need time to ask all their questions and absorb the responses. Experienced professionals understand these matters and respond fully and patiently. They know that properly informed parents are more likely to participate in and comply with the recommended treatment.

Coping With the Problem

The feelings and needs described above are common and quite normal, reflecting as they do the common challenges of living with an ADD child. Gaining an understanding of each family's particular emotional concerns by both professionals and the parents themselves is an essential goal of the treatment process. Most families are reassured when told that, even though there are no quick and sure cures for attention deficit disorder, a meaningful improvement in the child's behavior and its impact on the emotional health of the family is usually possible. This requires the parents' thorough understanding of ADD and its impact on each family member. It also requires that the parents gain renewed confidence in their own strengths, and in their ability to cope more effectively with their frustrations and uncertainty.

Identifying Parental Strengths

The first step in coping with the behavior of an ADD child (and the problems this creates within the family) is for parents to identify and deal with their own feelings toward the child. Many parents are capable of doing this type of self-analysis with little assistance. Others will benefit from the help of their support system of friends and extended family. An important goal for parents is to identify and build on the strengths and resources of their family when dealing with these problems.

Single parent families may find this particularly difficult. When these resources are exhausted, other help is needed such as contact with professionals, or other parents of ADD children. We will further discuss these helping strategies on pages 90 to 96.

Importance of Consistency and Predictability

As discussed earlier, an ADD child can have a very stressful impact on the family. Success in reducing this family stress depends significantly on how consistent parents are when dealing with their child's behavior, and how they determine and enforce rules. Parents who work as a team and agree upon rules and expectations have a greater probability of success when handling behavior management issues. Parents who disagree on rules and expectations undermine their spouse's efforts. They create confusion and unpredictability for the child, reducing their parental authority. In this atmosphere the child learns to play one parent against the other, thus increasing dissension and stress within the family. This reinforces the negative interaction cycle within the family and further diminishes family harmony. Successful parents generally agree upon realistic rules and obtainable goals. With these ideas in mind, they work towards gradual and steady improvement, rather than striving for instant perfection.

Parental Burn Out

Parents of ADD children commonly state, "We have tried everything but nothing works for any period of time. We always seem to be angry and find ourselves only responding to his bad behavior." It is difficult for parents to acknowledge and reinforce positive behavior when they are continually presented with behavioral challenges. Consequently, parents of ADD children often focus their attention on the child's poor behavior while ignoring appropriate conduct. They exhaust all their other behavior management strategies and rely only on one method – punishment. Eventually, they reach a point where they are physically and emotionally exhausted. They feel defeated and helpless. They are now experiencing "parental burn out," at which point they may be more susceptible to harming their child, physically and emotionally. At this point (preferably before) parents need professional help to cope with their problems.

Seeking Help and Meeting Professionals

Obtaining resources for the child and the family sometimes becomes a major responsibility for the parents. Communicating the family's needs and promoting their child's needs are often emotionally taxing experiences, especially if parents feel that they are being patronized and not given credit for their concerns. Often parents feel that their physician does not appreciate the depth of the family's distress and does not recognize his or her own inadequacy to deal with the family's problems. When parents feel a need for referral to another professional or a specialized agency, they may meet resistance. Services may be in short supply, waiting lists may be long and there may be concerns about financial costs. If this is the case, accessing resources and services in the community can become a major challenge for the family.

The parents' goal in dealing with professionals should be to promote a working alliance with them. Of course, this is also the goal of professionals in helping families. To achieve this goal the parents may find it helpful to utilize the following general strategies:

1. Prepare to meet a professional by having a specific goal or set of goals. Then focus on discussing your concerns. Do not talk about irrelevant and unrelated topics.

2. Allow the professional to address your concerns one at a time and answer his or her questions directly without wandering off on a tangent. Adopt a listening attitude. Remember, the experience of the professional in managing similar problems can work to your advantage.

3. Be cautious in criticizing other professionals in their handling of your child's problems. It is not improper to express these concerns but it is wise to do so in an open-minded and flexible way if possible.

4. Try not to label your child. Instead describe your impression of your child's problems. Leave the diagnosis to the professional who can come to a proper conclusion if problems are well described. If the situation improves, let the professional know. Positive feedback is important. If the problem continues or becomes worse, ask for another appointment to explore other possibilities. Treatment programs often need to be continuously monitored and modified. Make sure at the outset you learn how often the program is to be reviewed.

Resources for Parents and Families

Many families of ADD children do well in the care of their family physician only. Others will benefit from utilizing different resources in the community. What follows is a brief description of some resources for parents and families of ADD children. Unfortunately not all these resources are available in every community.

Parent Counselling

Professional parent counselling services are available in many communities. Parents can access these services through their family physicians, school counsellors or community health agencies. Parent counselling involves exploring parents' concerns regarding the troublesome behaviors of the ADD child, providing suggestions for behavioral management, promoting healthy self-esteem, and generally helping parents with communication and advocacy issues.

Parent Education Workshops

Periodic workshops for parents, teachers and others are organized in many communities to provide basic information about ADD, including the various forms of treatment available for it. If such workshops are not available in the community, parents can get assistance in organizing one by contacting the professional staff of the nearest centre which offers diagnostic and treatment services for ADD children and their families.

Family Therapy

While family therapy can take a number of different approaches, the goal of therapy is always to facilitate change in a caring and non-blaming way by utilizing various intervention techniques in a well-coordinated treatment plan. Family therapy for ADD children complements other forms of treatment. It involves the therapist meeting with the ADD child and his family to explore how the child's behavior affects each member of the family. The therapist also helps the family members utilize their strengths to cope with their emotions.

Family therapy usually requires several sessions. In the initial sessions the parents and siblings are allowed to express their feelings, their frustrations and anger. They are also encouraged to talk about the methods that they have tried to resolve their conflicts. Usually there are many issues. The therapist helps the family to establish priorities while setting realistic goals for change. Family members are encouraged to identify their strengths and the therapist capitalizes on these attributes while suggesting alternative, and hopefully more effective means of resolving conflicts. When parents notice recognizable (though small) changes in their family relationships, they will further support one another as a team. This strengthens the marital bond, restores their sense of competence in problem-solving and enhances their self worth. Whatever method of family therapy is used, families need to be understood and the focus of treatment should emphasize solutions that are effective.

ADD Parent Groups

Some communities have parent support groups for parents of ADD children. The objectives of these groups are the same as those of parent counselling or family therapy. The groups provide parents with support from other parents and professional group leaders. They offer an opportunity to discuss feelings and problems with others who are experiencing similar difficulties. Often parents share their methods of coping with the difficult behavior problems of ADD children.

At the Alberta Children's Hospital, the parent groups approach problem solving and decision making at their meetings and concentrate on:

- identification and clarification of issues
- development of alternative methods to deal with issues
- implementation of a plan of action
- evaluation of the outcome of these plans

The parents meet in eight weekly evening sessions with one or two group leaders and often continue meeting on an informal basis following these eight structured meetings. The groups are organized according to the age of the child, with one group being for parents of children nine and under and the other for parents of children ten years and older. This allows parents the opportunity to share their experiences and to gain the support and insight of others in the group who are raising children of comparable age.

In the first session the parents are encouraged to share both the challenges they face, and the resources they have found to be both supportive and helpful. We have found that, due to the intensity of their experiences, the ADD parent groups quickly develop into cohesive units. Initially it is difficult for parents to shift away from their negative thinking. However, with encouragement they are able to identify the positive elements (and opportunities) for learning and growth in parenting the ADD child. Once they start, they enthusiastically add to the list of the more positive aspects of parenthood. The words and phrases they use include: *challenging, creative, energetic, enthusiastic, empathetic, stronger, patient, involved, accessible, appreciative, assertive, determined, more aware of deficit, need to look for more positives, need to develop more parenting skills.*

In the sessions that follow parents are provided with information on the nature of ADD and its management. There are reviews of stimulant therapy, behavior therapy, diet and any other forms of management that they wish to discuss. This information helps the parents to clarify any misconceptions that they may have had. It improves their ability to interpret what they read in lay publications, or hear from their neighbors and friends. Most of all, it helps them to develop an ability to cope with the child's problems rather than seeking a cure.

Other sessions focus on the impact of the ADD child on family relationships. This includes the effects on extended family relationships, sibling relationships, and interactions both within and outside the family. Group facilitators often use techniques such as humor to reduce tension which enables parents to look back on stressful events in a comical light. Humor is an integral part of the therapeutic process. As entertainer Bill Cosby is reported to have said, "Most people don't realize it, but the key to survival as parents is retrospect; retrospect because they were once children and there lies 70% of the answers." In looking back some parents identify that they, or a family member, have had similar problems.

The ADD parent group program also includes topics pertaining to communication, self-esteem and behavior management. The specific agenda for the group is decided at the first meeting and modified in keeping with the needs of the group at later sessions. Parents contribute to the group process by working with others to find more effective problem-solving techniques which emerge from past successful experiences.

Behavior Management

Behavior management is usually a topic of the greatest interest for parents. Psychologists are frequently invited to these group sessions to discuss certain principles of child development and the approaches used in dealing with problem behaviors concurrent with the child's stage of emotional and intellectual maturity. Such group discussions often provide parents with fresh ideas and renewed enthusiasm to deal with the challenges of their child's behaviors.

Communication

Parents and teachers of ADD children are partners in the management of behavior. As such the parents' interaction with the school and the promotion of a positive working relationship with school personnel should be examined in a session. Parent-school interactions may evolve into conflict and mutual blaming. The complexity of the child's problems may not be well understood by the school personnel and as a result, the child may acquire new maladaptive behaviors in school. The situation can easily frustrate both the school and parents. The goal of this valuable session is for parents to develop more positive and productive methods of communicating with schools, and to solve problems co-operatively, whenever possible. An education consultant is brought in at this time to review with the parents the available local resources, and the appropriate lines of communication with schools and school boards.

The final session concerns parental self-care and program evaluation. Parents are encouraged to give feedback, share their feelings about the group process and identify areas which they felt were beneficial, as well as those which were not. Group leaders also give feedback in support of individual group members so as to maximize their potential in terms of problem-solving, self awareness and constructive decision making. Verbal feedback and completed questionnaires done by the parents are used to evaluate the content and the process of group sessions. This information is then used for planning future groups.

Our experience with parent support groups has convinced us that the groups are very effective as a supplemental mode of treatment. The groups help parents not only understand ADD, but also help them cope with their day-to-day stresses and difficulties. Initially, parents are concerned with their child and his behavior. As the sessions progress, the parents focus more on themselves, seeking out their previously unrecognized strengths to help their child. Parents report that as a result of this group experience they feel more in control when handling their ADD child and better able to communicate within the family. They also become more accepting of one another and more confident in their parenting roles.

Most importantly, the sessions give parents an opportunity to see that they are not alone. They learn that others experience similar feelings of isolation and frustration. Within an environment of acceptance and support, parents listen and learn from each others' stories and in many cases they leave feeling more hopeful about their ability to cope with present and future challenges.

9   Classroom Management

Well begun is half done.

– Aristotle, 384 - 322 B.C.

S. Gupta

Teaching a child with ADD is a major challenge for most teachers. In addition to the normal demands of the classroom, the teacher is required to deal with the disruptive, non-compliant behavior of the inattentive, impulsive child and to help him with his academic progress – a most difficult task indeed!

The principles of behavior management are outlined in Chapter 7 and are applicable both at home and at school. Normal school children learn strategies for successful learning and the rules of appropriate behavior with relative ease. ADD children, on the other hand, have to be taught how to organize their work, how to stay on task and complete assignments, learn why and how not to interrupt, and how to avoid conflict. The majority of teachers are familiar with techniques of assisting children to master these skills and use them effectively. Some teachers respond to the challenge of teaching an ADD child by improving their own teaching and interpersonal skills. A few find the presence of an ADD child in the classroom too disruptive and experience difficulty fulfilling the challenges and the special responsibilities of their profession. What follows is a brief outline of strategies that teachers may find useful in dealing with some common classroom problems encountered by ADD children.

Classroom Problems

A. The child daydreams, does not seem to listen and does not follow directions.

Most of us take the ability to listen for granted, since normal children have no difficulty doing so. Listening requires the ability to focus attention on what is being said and to ignore all other sights, sounds and thoughts which are irrelevant. This is precisely the skill that ADD children are lacking. This problem can be addressed in three stages: prelistening strategies, strategies that can be used during the listening process, and those which can be used after listening.

Prelistening strategies can be taught by making the purpose of the lesson completely clear. This can be done verbally and by outlining it on the board. The aim here is to strengthen the motivation to learn. The teacher must assure that the ADD child's attention is drawn to, and focused upon, the point and importance of the lesson. Periodic verbal reminders, or better still, agreed upon unspoken signals may be necessary for the ADD child to listen or to remain on-task. For example, if the child is not listening and is preoccupied with another activity, the teacher can walk over and gently touch his shoulder. However, teachers must decide on strategies that they are comfortable with and think will work. These may include a gesture, a word or a look. It is very important that the technique chosen does not embarrass or humiliate the child.

To encourage the development of listening skills, it is important that the teacher organize the information being presented. This can be done by highlighting what is going to be discussed. When the information presented is arranged according to time or sequence, it is less confusing for the ADD child and this facilitates his listening. ADD children, more than normal children, need to know not only what it is that they are required to learn, but also its relevance. This may be achieved by explicitly relating the vocabulary and concepts being taught to the child's interests and background experience. Half of the battle is won if the teacher can engage the child.

Postlistening skills can be taught by using the technique of verbal rehearsal with direct instruction such as: "Repeat in your own words . . . ;" and by using visual imagery, "Make a picture in your own head." These students can be encouraged to infer meaning by anticipating "why, how, what and where" questions.

Since ADD children find it very difficult to pay attention, it is important that the teacher present the instruction in a clear sequence and at a rate that is neither too slow nor too fast. Many ADD children cannot remember more than one or two instructions at a time and learn better when information is presented directly, rather than in a way which requires abstract deduction or discovery. In summary, it is very important that material be presented clearly, efficiently and in a way that catches the interest of the child. Once directions are given having the child repeat them softly to himself may help him remember. Reviewing the rules and prompting them should help to promote compliance.

ADD children often have difficulty in moving from one activity or class to another. Switching the object of their attention may be a particular challenge. They often need help in remembering rules at these times.

B. The child cannot start a task and complete it

To encourage on-task behavior and task completion the teacher can give reinforcement on a fixed schedule, that is, at regular intervals or after a set number of responses. Reinforcers are briefly discussed in Chapter 7 and include anything which tends to increase the frequency of a desired behavior. For example, verbal praise such as, "Good John, you worked two minutes quietly," encourages on-task behavior. If a child is doing a mathematics exercise, he should be asked to complete one or two problems only – not the entire sheet. When the child completes this portion, he is praised and asked to complete the next two problems. The teacher can gradually increase the size of each segment until the child learns to complete the entire task. In doing so, the teacher allows the child every opportunity to be successful.

It is important for the teacher to keep this principle in mind even when assigning homework. The amount of homework given should fit the child's attentional capacity.

C. The child is disruptive in the class

To deal with the disruptive behavior of an ADD child, the teacher can alter classroom seating arrangements. For example, place the child in front of and close to the teacher's desk, or next to a quiet highly motivated student. Ignoring as much of the disruptive behavior as possible sometimes helps to extinguish that behavior. The acknowledgement of an inappropriate behavior may be a reinforcer for an ADD child. Non-verbal cues that the teacher and ADD student have agreed upon can be used as a signal to help the child realize that what he is doing is not acceptable. The teacher may anticipate the child's behavior and prevent the problem with a quiet reminder. Often the teacher's presence is a deterrence to disruptive behavior. When the child makes noises, giggles, coughs, etc., the teacher can ask the child to run an errand or to perform some other chore in the classroom. This is a useful technique which allows the child to discontinue the disruptive behavior without embarrassment.

This is not, however, always effective. Nor is it convenient for the teacher to follow through with such techniques at all times. Clear, prompt and frequent feedback with appropriate consequences applied to the child's unacceptable behavior is effective. The nature and logic of these consequences, whether they be reinforcers or punishments must be more explicit for ADD children than for other children. Punishments such as response cost, losing privileges, or time out must be meaningful to the individual child. They will only be meaningful if the child values what he is about to lose. When incentives are used they must be reinforcing enough to motivate the child. Therefore, they must be selected carefully for the individual child and changed frequently. Teachers should aim to use "positives" before "negatives" as this helps to improve the attitude of the child and the overall atmosphere in the classroom.

D. The child has frequent temper tantrums

Tantrums have several stages and each must be dealt with differently. The first stage is the grumbling stage. The teacher usually recognizes a pattern of events which may lead to the child's tantrum. For example, the teacher may observe that the child becomes angry before or after a certain activity. She can help the child to verbalize his frustrations and this often prevents a full blown tantrum. Without drawing attention to the child, the teacher can walk over to him and say, "I think you are upset and I am wondering if ___ happened as you were walking in just now. Let's see how you can make it different for yourself so you are not upset."

The second stage in the tantrum is the noisy stage, when the child is aware of breaking the rules and is signalling for help. The child seems to be seeking external control. At this time it is necessary for the teacher not to say that the child is breaking the rules but to help him signal his wish for assistance in a more appropriate manner. The teacher may say, "I know you are angry. You can have quiet time for two minutes at your desk."

During the next stage the child has a full blown loss of composure. The child usually refuses to accept any suggestions the teacher may make. It may not be possible to manage his tantrum at this stage. It may be necessary to remove him from the classroom.

This is followed by the "leave me alone stage." It is best to leave the child alone and allow him to regain his control.

In the last stage, the child has regained control over his emotions. At this time the teacher can help the child to develop more effective problem solving skills. He can be helped to find answers to the following questions:

1. What was it that made you angry?
2. What did you expect to gain by doing what you did?

3. How could you have got what you wanted without getting so upset?

The use of these techniques is demanding and requires a great deal of patience and planning.

Cognitive Behavior Therapy

As stated in Chapter 7, the process of behavior modification involves a change of consequence and/or a restructuring of the environment *by others* in response to the inappropriate behavior of the ADD child. There can be a disadvantage in that the child may learn to become dependent on external controls to behave according to the expectations of the classroom or society.

On the other hand, cognitive behavior therapy teaches the child *self* control. The techniques of cognitive behavior therapy can also be used during classroom instruction. The child is taught to "think out loud" and use self-guiding verbalizations, self-monitoring and self-reinforcement in solving problems. Various components of cognitive behavioral therapy are outlined in Chapter 7 and will not be repeated here. The following examples should serve to demonstrate how this approach might be used in the classroom:

" *A boy bought five pieces of gum at 9¢ each. How much did he spend?* "

1. **What am I supposed to do?** I am supposed to know how much money the boy spent.
2. **What are the possibilities?** He spent more than 9¢ because he bought five pieces. I can either add or multiply.
3. **I must concentrate** on what is the best way of finding the answers.
4. **I must chose the right answer.** I think I will multiply.
5. **Self monitoring** – I think I did it right.

6. **Self reinforcement** – I did a good job because I thought it through. Or, I did not get the right answer. I will try harder the next time.

A similar approach can be used in teaching social skills. For example, Billy is knocked down by Joey in the playground. Billy's first impulse is to punch Joey. Instead he is taught to ask himself:

1. **What is the problem?** I am angry because Joey knocked me down.

2. **What can I do?** I can punch Joey, but that will get me into trouble. I can ignore Joey, but that is difficult and I remain angry. I can talk to the teacher and he can talk to Joey. Or, I can talk to Joey myself and tell him I don't like to be knocked down and will not put up with it in the future.

3. **Focusing attention.** I must think and choose the best answer to my problem.

4. **Choosing the best answer.** I think I will talk to Joey myself.

5. **Self reinforcement.** I am proud of myself for not allowing my anger to get me into trouble.

Such problem-solving approaches have been used in many school curriculum guides for teachers. A particularly useful one is *Elementary Mathematics Curriculum Guide* developed by the Alberta Department of Education. It consists of four basic steps: understanding the problem, developing a plan, carrying out the plan, and looking back at the plan. Within each step are problem solving strategies which assist in the thinking through and solving of problems. These strategies are outlined in the following table. Not all of these strategies are suitable for students in the earlier grades. Interested teachers should consult this curriculum guide for grade-by-grade treatment.

Problem Solving: Integral to all Mathematics

Grade Level 6

General Learner Expectations	Related Specific Learner Expectations	Developmental Span (by school years)						
		P	1	2	3	4	5	6
The student applies a variety of strategies in solving problems related to concepts from the strands, uses the stages in solving a problem, and justifies the solution process.	**Demonstrating traits of a good problem solver**							
	The student:							
	– demonstrates a willingness to find a solution to the problem							→
	– perseveres in finding a solution to the problem							→
	– demonstrates flexibility in finding solutions to problems							→
	– presents ideas in an understandable way							→
	– works both independently and in a group							→
	Understanding the problem							
	The student:							
	– understands words and phrases							→
	– understands the questions asked							→
	– identifies given information							→
	– interprets pictures and diagrams							→
	– restates the problem in own words							→
	– understands what information is implied							→
	– understands what information is missing							→
	– understands what information is extraneous							→

Developing and carrying out a plan

The student:
- uses logical reason (process of elimination)
- acts it out
- uses manipulatives and trial-and-error
- looks for and continues patterns
- draws pictures and diagrams
- collects and uses data (tally, pictographs, bar graphs, stem-and-leaf plots and line graphs)
- chooses and carries out the appropriate operation using an appropriate method (paper-and-pencil, mental calculation, or calculator)
- does a simpler but related problem
- guesses and checks
- uses tables or lists
- works backwards
- monitors the process in carrying out the plan

Looking back

The student:
- states the answer(s) to the problem
- determines if the answer is reasonable
- discusses the solution process with others
- retells the problem with the solution
- looks for other ways to solve the problem
- does similar problems
- alters the problem and finds the effect
- generalizes the solution
- creates problems that exemplify the concepts learned

Elementary Mathematics Curriculum Guide, 1993 (Draft)

Alberta Education, Edmonton, Alberta

10 Other Approaches to Management

Men willingly believe what they wish

– Julius Caesar, 100 - 44 B.C.

Diet and Hyperactivity

In the 1970s, the protest movement concerning the "drugging" of school children was still quite vocal. During the same period, the "back-to-nature" movement was also gaining momentum. The time was right for the introduction of a different approach to the management of ADD which, in spite of the effectiveness of stimulant therapy, remained a major challenge for all professionals. Dr. Ben Feingold of San Francisco, impressed by the successful treatment of aspirin-sensitive adults with a diet which was free of naturally-occurring salicylates (aspirin or ASA is acetylsalicylic acid), hypothesized that hyperactive and learning-disabled children might also respond to this treatment. Clinical experience had shown that tartrazine a yellow food coloring and aspirin could induce identical clinical problems in aspirin-sensitive individuals, even though the two substances are not chemically or structurally related. In some patients, the exclusion of foods which contained naturally-occurring salicylates did not improve their clinical picture but when tartrazine was also excluded, it did. However, some patients continued to have problems, even when on a diet free of both naturally-occurring salicylates and tartrazine. Dr. Feingold then hypothesized that, since literally thousands of food colorings, flavorings and preservatives are added to our foods during processing, some of them (though chemically not related to tartrazine or aspirin) might be responsible for the clinical picture of aspirin sensitivity. This was the basis for the introduction of Dr. Feingold's K-P diet (named after Kaiser-Permanente Medical Centre, where Dr. Feingold worked), which was salicylate and additive free. He claimed that a number of conditions involving many body organs and systems were manifestations of adverse reactions to some naturally occurring substances in food and / or food additives. He further hypothesized that adverse reactions occur only in certain genetically-predisposed, sensitive individuals.

Dr. Feingold initially claimed that a large number of hyperactive and learning disabled children responded to the K-P diet, and that they showed a marked deterioration in their behavior following the re-introduction of the offending foods. In 1975 he published his well-known and popular book, *Why Your Child is Hyperactive*. The timing of this book was perfect. Following its publication many parents and professionals, including many physicians who objected to stimulant therapy, resorted to using the K-P diet. Since that time, all professionals working with hyperactive children have heard many stories of disappointment, as well as dramatic improvement, in the behavior of some hyperactive children following dietary modifications.

The history of medicine is replete with claims of success in the treatment of all sorts of ailments. Medical scientists however have learned not to accept anecdotal or testimonial evidence until its validity is scientifically demonstrated. There is nothing wrong with anecdotes or testimonials. They are the initial observations which form the impetus for all scientific inquiries. Scientists draw inferences based on their observations and then propose more formal hypotheses which may be tested. To evaluate their hypotheses they set up experiments which may either prove or discredit them. In medicine, claims of treatment success are subjected to rigorous tests before they are either accepted as useful, or rejected. Throughout the history of science, and particularly during the twentieth century, scientists have become increasingly sophisticated in their design of experiments (clinical trials). The experimental studies done on the effectiveness of various treatments of ADD are examples of this sophistication.

We can all be biased "for" or "against" any form of treatment. Our bias can influence our observations. Therefore, experimental studies must be designed in such a way as to minimize the bias. Double-blind methods, using active and inactive (placebo) treatments, in which neither the investigators nor the persons who are being treated know the form of treatment being given, are the cornerstone of these experimental designs.

When the effectiveness of a drug is being investigated, it is relatively easy to produce a placebo with the same size, shape, color and taste to counteract the influence of bias. Investigation of the effectiveness of dietary modifications is not that easy. How does one prevent the child from raiding the refrigerator or the cookie jar? How does one ensure that the child does not eat a candy, or something else, given to him by his friends? How does one hide the color or taste of foods, if food colorings, flavor enhancers, or food preservatives are removed from or added to the child's food? These are a few of many difficulties which must be overcome in studying diet and its relationship to behavior. Many techniques have been developed to do so. These include the removal of all foods from the home and supplying the family's entire food requirement for several weeks. During this time the composition of the diet is altered without the family's knowledge.

Almost all of these studies have been criticized for "methodological flaws," that is, imperfections in the study designs which make it difficult to draw valid conclusions from them. Furthermore, in scientific circles, the results of even the most well-designed studies are often not readily accepted, until similar results are duplicated by other researchers elsewhere. To this point, a few well-designed studies have demonstrated that some ADD children show a modest improvement in their behavior following dietary modifications and that this improvement does not appear to be a placebo effect. Our own studies of hyperactive preschool children have demonstrated similar results. Unfortunately no one can predict which child may benefit from dietary modifications. Current research in a number of centres indicates that there is a tremendous variability in children's response to foods. In practice, the experience of most physicians, children and families has been that the benefits of changing the diet (in comparison to other treatments) are negligible, or so small, that the inconvenience and expense of the new diet does not warrant the change. A great deal of research is still required to clarify the many unanswered questions regarding the effects of diet and dietary modification on children's behavior.

Since the introduction of the K-P diet, panels of experts, consisting of well known researchers from many fields in the United States, have reviewed the evidence derived from studies concerning the relationship between diet and selective attention. Their conclusions have been similar. Further research is required to prove the existence of any relationship between diet and attention. Of course this does not mean that there is no relationship between food and human behavior. It merely means that the relationship between food additives, or naturally-occurring substances in food and the behavior of ADD children has not been conclusively demonstrated.

Despite this scientific conclusion some parents remain convinced that their children have benefited from the K-P diet. Many other parents inquire about similar dietary modifications for their children. Since *additive-free* diets have not been associated with any harmful effects, there is no reason to discourage families who wish to pursue such a diet. Diets which are free of *naturally-occurring salicylates*, however, are very restrictive and can result in nutritional deficiencies if they are not under the supervision of a trained dietitian. Parents must ensure that their children are receiving the recommended minimum daily amounts of essential nutrients. It is imperative that parents consult their family physicians or pediatricians before embarking on this type of diet. Many physicians remain opposed to dietary modification for the treatment of ADD and will advise against it. If, in spite of the advice of their physicians, parents wish to pursue this diet, they can obtain assistance regarding their child's nutritional requirements from their local health departments. The local associations for children and adults with learning disabilities may also provide some help.

Dr. Feingold has published a second book, *The Feingold Cookbook for Hyperactive Children* which parents may find useful. It must be emphasized that it is difficult to give any restrictive diet of this nature to only one member of the family. Usually the diet of the entire family must be changed and this may cause the family considerable inconvenience and expense.

The relationship between behavior and certain neurotransmitters in the brain was mentioned earlier (pp. 29, 32 to 33). There are a few studies which show that increasing certain normal dietary components, which are the precursors (building blocks) of these neurotransmitters, increases their concentration in the brain. Since the therapeutic effectiveness of this type of dietary modification has not been demonstrated, this approach to treatment cannot be recommended at this time.

Sugar and Hyperactivity

Many parents also claim dramatic improvements in their children's behavior when sugar intake is restricted. Again, this is testimonial evidence which has provided an impetus for scientific research. Blinded studies carried out on the effect of sugar on children's behavior have demonstrated only the placebo effect of this treatment. In other words, when mothers are blind to the experiment (i.e., they do not know whether the child is receiving sugar or an artificial sweetener in his food or drink), their rating of the child's behavior does not correspond to what the child is actually taking.

A recent well-designed double-blind study on the effect of acute (one time) sugar load versus artificial sweeteners on the behavior of ADD and normal children did not reveal any increase in *aggressive* behavior of either group of children.

There was, however, a noticeable decrease in the *attention span* of ADD children. The scientists of this study issued a caution regarding the interpretation of their results, since all children were between the ages of 5½ and 7½ years, which is considered to be the borderline age suitable for testing the attention span with their test material (named *Continuous Performance Task*). The authors of this study recommend replication of their study with older children.

Once again, since sugar is not an essential component of the human diet, we cannot discourage parents who wish to pursue a low sugar diet for their children from doing so. More rational advice regarding sugar, food additives and a salicylate-free diet can be given only when future research clarifies many as yet unanswered questions.

Megavitamin Therapy

There are some individuals with genetic deficits who, in order to function normally, require greater amounts of certain nutrients than is required by most people. A number of uncommon disorders are known to fall into this category. Some scientific observers have suggested that some disturbances of brain function might also be caused by a nutrient "deficiency." For example, there are claims that megavitamin therapy is useful in the treatment of schizophrenia. This proposal still has its supporters, despite the fact that carefully designed scientific research has failed to prove its effectiveness. Some researchers have postulated that ADD could be caused by a genetically-determined increased need for some vitamins. Once again, well-conducted scientific research has not proven the efficacy of megavitamin therapy in the management of ADD. In fact, a recent study demonstrated adverse effects of large doses of some water-soluble vitamins, which until now have been considered relatively harmless. For this reason, megavitamin therapy should be avoided until further research has clearly demonstrated its efficacy and safety in children when used over prolonged periods of time.

It must be emphasized that when the child is given any form of treatment, whether it be stimulant therapy, K-P diet, low sugar diet, or megavitamin therapy, the benefits and potential harmful side-effects for the child and his family must be carefully considered. Some forms of treatment may harm the child by depriving him of a more effective means of treatment. Other forms of treatment may create a great deal of family stress. This may be the case when, for the benefit of the affected child, the entire family is placed on a diet which may be costly, inconvenient, or unpalatable to the entire family.

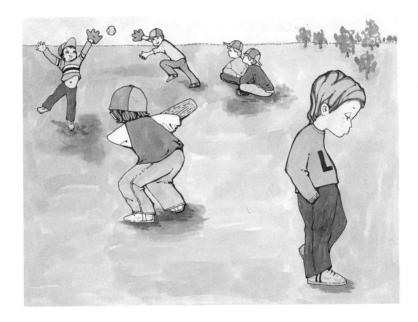

11   ADD in Adolescence

*For God's sake, give me the young man who has brains enough
to make a fool of himself.*

– Robert Louis Stevenson, 1850 - 1894

Joel Fagan M.D. & Carolyn Garbett-Smith, MSW

Adolescents experience rapid changes in physical, psychological, sexual and social development. At this time, the adolescent experiences "growth spurts," puberty and a strong need to be independent from parents. Developing maturity is often defined in terms of tasks, such as becoming independent, expanding the number of relationships outside the home and forming a value system appropriate to adult life. Most people successfully accomplish these developmental tasks by age 25. Adolescents are expected to gradually gain control over behaviorial impulses, with suitable expression of their sexual drives. All of these changes ultimately allow the individual to choose a successful life path, which includes appropriate employment and stable social relationships.

Adolescence is also a time when school responsibilities can be very stressful. Throughout this portion of their education, expectations increase and the student is expected to develop organizational skills, good study habits and creative thinking. With each higher grade the demands upon selective attention increase. Therefore, it is not surprising that most of us consider our teenage years to have been quite challenging, both for ourselves and our families.

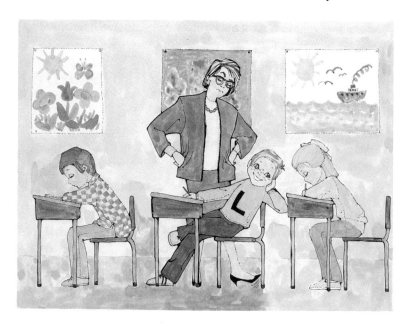

Adolescents with ADD

When an adolescent has ADD these challenges and re-sponsibilities become even more of a problem. Long term difficulties in achieving success hinders both self confidence and independence. ADD adolescents have difficulties in de-veloping control over cravings and drives because of their ongoing impulsiveness and difficulty in learning from past experiences. Faulty judgement and weak social skills impede the growth of relationships within and beyond the family. Weak selective attention creates a barrier to academic success and career planning. All of these factors add further stress to the parent-adolescent relationship.

Taking medication may be actively questioned by adoles-cents. The majority will experience uncomfortable emotions concerning this form of treatment at some point. Some will question the safety of medication, perhaps fearing addiction or other health complications. Many will worry about the effect on their reputation if their friends know they are taking medicine to help learning and behavior. Some will take exception to certain side effects of stimulant drugs, such as reduced appetite or sleep problems. Many others will feel a type of stress, difficult for them to describe, which is the result of inner conflict between their need for independence and their need for medication. The need for independence in thought and action is a universal concern among teenagers. This need may be expressed by them in a wish to be independent of having ADD and needing treatment, aswell as of parents and teachers who are seeking their cooperation. When faced with these emotions, it is not uncommon for adolescents to decide to stop their medication, despite the wishes of their parents and teachers.

The situation at home and at school usually worsens when treatment is discontinued at a time when it remains necessary and helpful. Grades may fall, friendships may be further damaged and family relationships become further strained. Since emotional stress in itself will further weaken selective attention (worsen ADD), the overall situation may quickly deteriorate.

Treatment for the Adolescent with ADD

Parents or teachers who recognize the adolescent's resistance to taking medication should seek professional help promptly, particularly if their own efforts are not effective in resolving the problem. The longer a period of turmoil lasts, the more difficult it may be for the professional to reestablish productive communication with – and effective treatment of – the adolescent. If the adolescent has fears about the safety of medication, simple reassurance may be sufficient. When there is concern about others knowing about the need for drug therapy, the sustained release kinds of medication (see pages 58 to 59), which eliminate the need to take the medicine at school, may solve the problem.

Where the adolescent is in emotional conflict concerning independence versus the ADD and drug treatment, the professional is well advised at the outset to explain that these feelings are common and natural and do not mean that the adolescent is behaving badly. Treatment decisions are difficult when such feelings exist. The professional should do everything possible to guide the young person through what is essentially an adult decision making process. The individual should be helped to compare the known personal benefits of medication with the equally valid, perceived disadvantages or side effects of the drugs. The professional should avoid becoming unduly judgemental or to actively take sides with any member of the family regardless of the treatment decision chosen. Rather, every effort should be made to respect this decision and to make it as easy as possible for all members the family, particularly the adolescent, to return in the future if circumstances change. Some may decide to stop their medication for a month or two, only to change their mind when their problems increase. If this happens, it is much better if the adolescent feels that the professional is sympathetic, approachable and respectful.

It should be emphasized that not all adolescents run into serious problems. In the majority of cases many of the problems which are part of ADD will gradually improve with increasing maturity. By the later years of high school selective attention itself will be stronger than in earlier years. With growing insight and experience the majority of young people will be able to deal with their problems in more effective ways. Many will learn how, when and where to study in order to get the best results. Also, at this time of life there are more choices available in study courses which allow individuals to better match their interests and abilities. In addition many of the symptoms of ADD which in earlier years caused great conflict will often improve during adolescence. These include hyperactivity, impulsiveness, moodiness and discipline problems. Nevertheless, difficulties with concentration and impulse control continue to be a concern for many people with ADD into their adult years.

By age 17 or 18 at least half of the people who needed medication in childhood will have stopped their treatment with their doctor's approval. The remainder (including many who continue their studies beyond high school) will continue to be treated safely and effectively into their adult years. In many communities there are relatively few physicians who have the training and experience to treat adult patients with ADD. This situation is gradually improving. A shortage of resources exists in most areas for the full range of services needed by adults with attention problems and learning disabilities. Information concerning available resources can usually be obtained through the local learning disabilities association.

The Newly Diagnosed Adolescent

When the diagnosis of ADD is first made during adolescence, the majority of patients experience mixed feelings. On one hand they may feel relief that their problem is recognized and there is hope of effective management. On the other hand they often have difficulty accepting the diagnosis and the need for any treatment. Physicians and other professionals should explain all aspects of ADD to the adolescent, and his or her parents, in terms which are understandable and in a manner which makes the young person feel like a partner in all treatment decisions. The benefits and side effects of medication should be thoroughly described. When this is accomplished, the chances increase that all family members will be comfortable in cooperating with the treatment program.

Following the onset of treatment some adolescents have described the improvement in their situation in interesting and revealing statements:

"Before taking my medication I had a storm in my head. Now all is calm."

"Before taking my pills it was like I was watching television with several programs on the screen at the same time. I couldn't pay attention to any one of them long enough to get the meaning out of it. Now there is only one program on at a time."

"Before, my own thoughts and ideas kept interfering with what was happening in school. I kept tuning out at the wrong time. Now I can concentrate on what the teacher is saying, and I can learn a lot easier."

For most people affected by ADD it is far preferable if their ADD is recognized and treated before they reach their teenage years. The longer young people struggle to achieve academic and social success, the harder it will be for all members of the treatment team, including the family and the adolescent, to reverse the effects of this long term problem. Even so, many parents of adolescents find it useful to participate in parent support groups. Teachers and school counsellors should be actively involved in efforts to support these students. In some cases adolescents may need individual counselling to help them cope with the emotional impact of their problems. In extreme situations, when the adolescent approaches a personal crisis because of long term social and academic failure, parents may experience immense anxiety over their child possibly committing suicide. Prompt mental health support should be obtained when these fears exist. Unfortunately, some unfounded statements by the press and others, have linked suicide in ADD adolescents with stimulant medications such as Ritalin. It must be emphatically stated that this concern is completely unfounded. Suicide in young people, when it is considered or attempted, is the result of despair and hopelessness. The causes of these depressed feelings arise from severe and prolonged failure and conflict which is commonly seen in untreated or inadequately treated ADD patients. These emotions are not the result of the medications used to treat the ADD.

Both parents and adolescents have many questions concerning prognosis and long term prospects for individuals with ADD. These questions are considered in chapter 12. Prospects are best if the adolescent continues to receive treatment as long as it is needed and when parents and teachers have a good understanding of the ADD problems and their impact on the affected individual.

12   When ADD Children Grow Up

The wildest colts make the best horses.

— Themistocles, 512 - 499 B.C.

Outcome Studies

There are many published studies on the outcome of childhood hyperactivity and ADD in adolescence and adulthood. Most of these studies suffer from limitations which are associated with all long-term follow-up studies and which make it difficult to draw valid conclusions from them. These limitations include the following:

1. ADD children are a mixed group of individuals. In some, hyperactivity is a prominent feature. In others it is less pronounced or absent. Some ADD children are highly intelligent, others are less intelligent. Some have understanding and patient parents, others do not. Some have been treated adequately, others less so. They all have had different upbringing. If all ADD children are combined in one group for outcome studies, it is difficult to interpret the results of this research since each subgroup of children may have a different prognosis.

In addition, most of the older follow-up studies did not use the diagnostic criteria proposed by the American Psychiatric Association. Thus it is difficult to compare the results of the older investigations with the more recent studies which apply these standards.

2. One of the most troublesome aspects of outcome studies is the lack of information about the segment of the ADD population lost to follow-up. Follow-up studies are usually done on children attending hospital-based clinics. Some ADD children and their families do not keep their return clinic appointments a few months or so after their initial assessment. If those ADD children who are responsive to treatment and faithfully return to clinics are the only ones included in outcome studies, one cannot be sure that the conclusions drawn from these studies can be applied to all ADD children. Those who are lost to follow-up are not necessarily similar to those who are followed; they may be different with respect to their initial symptoms, their intelligence, the strength of their families and many other factors which might influence their prognosis.

3. Another troublesome problem in outcome studies is that we do not know how well ADD children and their families follow through with their recommended treatment. In one study of compliance with the drug therapy, the children's urine was tested for the presence of the prescribed drugs. A large percentage of urine samples showed no trace of the prescribed medications. If we do not know how well the ADD children and their families follow through with recommended treatment, it is meaningless to draw conclusions from outcome studies about the differences between those who were apparently treated and those who were not.

4. The length of treatment of ADD children obviously affects their prognosis. In outcome studies further difficulties arise because many ADD children who take their medications more or less faithfully, do so for only a few years. They discontinue their medication either on the recommendation of their physicians or on their own initiative. This is because many ADD children are no longer hyperactive in their adoles-

cence and adulthood, even though they may continue having impulsiveness and attentional problems. Many outcome studies on the effectiveness of stimulant therapy have found that ADD children have a poor prognosis in terms of educational achievement and social adjustment. These findings should be interpreted with caution. If stimulant therapy is discontinued only because hyperactivity is no longer a major problem, the persistence of impulsiveness and attentional problems into adulthood cannot be attributed to the ineffectiveness of this form of treatment. One cannot conclude that ADD has an inherently poor prognosis. It can only be said that short-term stimulant therapy is ineffective in permanently eliminating impulsiveness and attentional problems. In other words, some ADD children require treatment for their inattention and impulsiveness in their adolescence and adulthood, even if they are no longer hyperactive. Without their medications they may continue to experience academic and social problems.

Many of these past outcome studies suggested a gloomy future for ADD children, predictings that they would not fare well as adults. Frequently, disappointment was expressed about the lack of long-term value of stimulant therapy, despite its obvious short-term benefits. This disappointment was based on the false expectation that stimulants would cure the disorder, or with maturation ADD children would outgrow their problems. Some of these initial studies indicated that aggression in ADD children was an indicator of a poor prognosis, since about one half of the aggressive ADD children developed antisocial problems in their adolescence. These studies do not tell us why the other half of aggressive ADD children did not develop antisocial problems. Nor do they tell us what happened to many aggressive ADD children who were lost to follow-up. Many of these studies also did not follow ADD children long enough to know what happened to them in adulthood.

With these limitations in mind we can now look at some of the better outcome studies. One of the more comprehensive studies has been carried out by investigators at the Montreal Children's Hospital. They have published the results of an ongoing five, ten and fifteen year follow-up study of several groups of hyperactive children seen in their clinic – quite a significant achievement. Since the symptom which identified this group of people was hyperactivity, they likely had a number of underlying causes for this problem. In other words, not all would be diagnosed as having ADD by today's standards. Their studies included information obtained from the affected individuals, their parents, teachers, school counsellors and employers. They also obtained psychiatric interviews, intelligence measurements, and documented certain aspects of the physical examination including height, weight, pulse and blood pressure. As might be expected, over the long period of this research their loss to follow-up was quite high. 15 years following the initial assessment only 61 of the original group of 104 individuals were available for study. Nevertheless, their results are interesting, and for many individuals quite encouraging.

Their five year follow-up group included 22 children who were treated with *chlorpromazine* (a tranquillizer) for 18 months to five years, 24 children who were treated with *methylphenidate* (Ritalin) for three to five years, and 22 affected children who received no treatment. There was no significant difference between these three groups in measurements of emotional adjustment, delinquency, or intelligence. However, those children who were treated with *methylphenidate* (Ritalin) were more manageable at home and at school.

The ten year follow-up study described 75 hyperactive children and 45 normal (non-hyperactive) children who served as a comparison or control group. The hyperactive children had received a number of different medications, for varying intervals and some had received individual counselling from a mental health professional. Unfortunately, the investigators concluded that, "In general, this group represented a relatively untreated group, with few receiving adequate counselling or drug therapy." This ten year follow-up compared a relatively untreated group of hyperactive children (by today's standards) with a group of normal children of similar age. After ten years the original 75 hyperactive children could be divided into three subgroups of young adults. The first, consisting of nearly 50% of the original group, had outgrown their symptoms and were functioning normally. The second subgroup, which was comparable in size to the first, continued to have significant problems with hyperactivity, impulsiveness and low self-esteem which interfered in varying degrees with their work and personal relationships. The third subgroup was a small statistically insignificant one whose members showed character or personality disorders. It should be stated again that these were young adults who as children were hyperactive and did not receive adequate treatment.

In comparison, in a separate 10 to 12 year follow-up study, these investigators compared 20 hyperactive children, who had received at least three years of treatment with *methylphenidate* (a relatively better, but still inadequately treated group) with normal controls. In many areas of life, including school, work and social relationships, the treatment group had experienced significantly more problems than the controls. In other areas, such as car accidents, delinquency, and a more positive view of their childhood, the more adequately treated hyperactive individuals actually did better than their untreated counterparts.

The 15 year follow-up included 61 of the original 104 hyperactive children and 41 of 45 normal controls. The results indicated that about 50% of the former group continued to have disabling life problems, which varied in severity from mild to very serious. 23 % reported some features of an antisocial personality disorder. It should be understood that this was based on self-administered questionnaires completed by adults, who as children were hyperactive. They did not all have antisocial behavior! Schizophrenia, alcoholism, and drug abuse did not occur more commonly in the hyperactive group.

In general, those who had antisocial behavior at the 15 year follow-up were continuing a pattern which began in earlier life. However, not all who showed this trait as children continued to do so as adults. The antisocial behavior seemed to result from the cumulative and prolonged interaction between a number of unfortunate factors, including: an aggressive personality, lower IQ, family poverty and mental health problems in other family members. Each of these adds to the burden of stress experienced by the ADD affected person. Among other things, this underscores the importance of an understanding and supportive family in influencing the outcome of the ADD adult.

It is very important to remember that many of the so-called "treated" individuals in the Montreal study did not receive adequate treatment. Would there be any difference between the controls and hyperactive individuals, if the latter group had received adequate treatment for as long as their symptoms persisted? This cannot be answered by the Montreal follow-up study.

The Montreal investigators have published their entire study, including a comprehensive literature review on this subject, in a book entitled *Hyperactive Children Grown Up* (see the Suggested Readings section).

Other long term follow-up studies have been reported by investigators from the United States and other countries. Even though this research does not provide definitive answers because of limitations in study design, the results reveal convincing trends. By early adulthood ADD appears to remain present in at least one third of subjects. Those with ADD in childhood do not have more psychiatric problems than those in the control group in adolescence and early adulthood, provided they had normal intelligence, and no additional disabilities or emotional disorders. Those with mental retardation, serious learning disabilities and severe mental health disorders have a much less favorable outlook. This emphasizes the need for early and comprehensive support services for this high risk group. Among adults with ongoing symptoms of ADD, their outlook can in many instances be favorably influenced by continuing their treatment as long as necessary.

The best hope for people with ADD of all ages lies in the early recognition of the problem, and prompt, comprehensive and long term treatment, often continued into adolescence and beyond. The following story should inspire those of us who prefer to remain optimistic:

According to the theory of aerodynamics, and as may be readily demonstrated through laboratory tests and wind tunnel experiments, the bumblebee is unable to fly. This is because the size, weight and shape of his body in relation to the total wing spread makes flying impossible. But the bumble bee, being ignorant of these profound scientific truths, goes ahead and flies anyway . . . and manages to make a little honey everyday!

Suggested Readings

For a more detailed discussion of the topics in this book, the readers may refer to the following books.

Becker, W. C. *Parents are Teachers*. Champaign, Illinois: Research Press, 1971.

Briggs, D. C. *Your Child's Self- Esteem*. New York: Dolphin Books, Doubleday and Co., 1975.

Copeland, Edna D. *Medications for Attention Disorders and Related Medical Problems: A Comprehensive Handbook*. Atlanta, GA: SPI Press, 1991.

Elementary Mathematics Curriculum Guide, 1982. Edmonton, Alberta: Alberta Education, 1993.

Goldstein, Sam & Goldstein, Michael. *Hyperactivity: Why Won't My Child Pay Attention*. New York: John Wiley and Sons, 1992.

Ingersoll, Barbara D. & Goldstein, Sam. *Attention Deficit Disorder and Learning Disabilities: Realities, Myths and Controversial Treatments*. New York: Doubleday, 1993.

Kendall, P. C. and Braswell, L. *Cognitive-Behavioral Therapy for Impulsive Children*. New York: Guilford Press, 1985.

Levine, M. D., Brooks, R. and Shonkoff, J. P. *A Pediatric Approach to Learning Disorders*. New York: John Wiley and Sons, 1980.

Levine, M. D. *Explaining Attention Deficits to Children: The Concentration Cockpit*. Cambridge, MA: Educators Publishing Service, 1987.

Sleator, E. K. and Pelham, W. E. Jr. *Attention Deficit Disorder*. Norwalk, Connecticut: Appleton-Century-Croft, 1986

Swift, M. S. and Spivack, G. *Alternative Teaching Strategies: Helping Behaviorally Troubled Children*. Champaigne, Illinois: Research Press, 1975.

Weiss, G. and Hechtman, L. T. *Hyperactive Children Grown Up: ADHD in Children, Adolescents, and Adults*. 2nd Edition. New York: Guilford Press, 1993.